The Role of
Pharmacoeconomics
in Outcomes
Management

NELDA E. JOHNSON, PharmD
DAVID B. NASH, MD
EDITORS

American Hospital Publishing, Inc.
An American Hospital Association Company
Chicago

This publication is designed to provide accurate and authoritative information in regard to the subject matter covered. It is sold with the understanding that neither the authors nor the publisher is engaged in rendering legal, accounting, or other professional service. If legal advice or other expert assistance is required, the services of a competent professional person should be sought.

The views expressed in this publication are strictly those of the authors and do not necessarily represent official positions of the American Hospital Association.

Library of Congress Cataloging-in-Publication Data

The role of pharmacoeconomics in outcomes management / edited by Nelda E. Johnson and David B. Nash.
     p.   cm.
    Includes bibliographical references and index.
    ISBN 1-55648-169-1
    1. Chemotherapy—Economic aspects. 2. Outcome assessment (Medical care) I. Johnson, Nelda E. II. Nash, David B.
    [DNLM: 1. Economics, Pharmaceutical. 2. Outcome Assessment (Health Care)   QV 736 R745 1996]
RM263.R65   1996
338.4'33621782—dc20
DNLM/DLC
for Library of Congress   96-35331
                                 CIP

Catalog no. 169111

©1996 by American Hospital Publishing, Inc.,
an American Hospital Association company

Printed in the USA

AHA is a service mark of the American Hospital Association used under license by American Hospital Publishing, Inc.

Text set in Trump

3M—12/96—0450

Audrey Kaufman, Senior Editor
Lisa Weder, Editor
Peggy DuMais, Assistant Manager, Production
Marcia Bottoms, Director, Books Division

Contents

About the Editors

Nelda E. Johnson, PharmD, is project director for health policy and clinical outcomes at Thomas Jefferson University Hospital, Inc., in Philadelphia. Her extensive experience includes hospital pharmacy practice, developing and supervising clinical pharmacy programs, conducting pharmacoeconomics and outcomes research, as well as teaching health care professionals to conduct their own research. Dr. Johnson is on the editorial board for the international publication *Pharmaco-Economics and Outcomes News* and writes a quarterly column on outcomes for the journal *Pharmacy & Therapeutics.* She is also a founder of the Association for Pharmacoeconomics and Outcomes Research (APOR) and works actively with pharmaceutical organizations, including the American Society of HealthSystem Pharmacists (ASHP) and the American College of Clinical Pharmacy (ACCP), to disseminate information about health economics and outcomes research. She has also assisted these organizations in the development of accreditation standards for fellowship programs in pharmacoeconomics and outcomes.

David B. Nash, MD, MBA, FACP, a board-certified internist, has been the first director, Office of Health Policy and Clinical Outcomes at Thomas Jefferson University and an associate professor of medicine at Jefferson Medical College in Philadelphia since 1990. Nationally recognized for his work in outcomes management, medical staff development, and quality-of-care improvement, his publications have appeared in three dozen articles in major journals and in five edited books. In 1995, he was awarded the Clifton Latiolais Prize by the American Managed Care Pharmacy Association. Dr. Nash received his BA in economics (Phi Beta Kappa) from Vassar College in New York and his MD from the University of Rochester School of Medicine and Dentistry.

He earned his MBA in health administration with honors from the Wharton School at the University of Pennsylvania. He is also a former Robert Wood Johnson Foundation clinical scholar and medical director of a nine-physician faculty group practice in general internal medicine.

About the Contributors

Sara J. Beis, RPh, MS, is a drug information specialist in the Henry Ford Health System in Detroit. She also serves as a member of the System's Ambulatory Care Formulary Committee. Ms. Beis provides pharmacoeconomic analysis to aid the formulary committee in drug therapy selection. She is one of the founders of the Association for Pharmacoeconomics and Outcomes Research (APOR). She frequently lectures on pharmacoeconomics and outcomes research to regional pharmacy groups. Additionally, Ms. Beis has extensive experience in drug therapy management and health care administration and has worked as a clinical pharmacist in inpatient, outpatient, and nursing home settings. Her administrative activities have included positions as an administrator of a medical group practice as well as acting chief of pharmacy services in the Veterans Administration System.

Joseph E. Biskupiak, PhD, MBA, is the director of Technology Assessment for Hastings Strategic Advantage, a division of Hastings Healthcare Group in Pennington, NJ. In this capacity he directs research in the areas of clinical outcomes, health service utilization, disease management, and clinical studies. Before joining Hastings, Dr. Biskupiak served as research assistant professor and assistant project director for the Office of Health Policy and Clinical Outcomes in the department of medicine at Thomas Jefferson University in Philadelphia. Dr. Biskupiak's responsibilities included assisting new businesses in health care policy development and conducting research in the areas of pharmacoeconomics, technology assessment, and health policy.

Becky Briesacher, BA, MA, is manager of the Institute for Pharmaceutical Economics at the Philadelphia College of Pharmacy and Science. She also serves as preceptor for several post-graduate pharmacoeconomic fellowships and as an adjunct faculty member. In addition, Ms. Briesacher is a senior associate of the Technology Assessment and Pharmacoeconomics Services Center of Excellence (a research collaboration with Thomas Jefferson University). Her research, publications, and lectures over the last four years have included measuring patient outcomes and quality of care in managed care with an emphasis on health insurance claims databases.

Caryl E. Carpenter, MPh, PhD, is an associate professor and chair of the department of health and medical services administration at Widener University in Chester, PA. Dr. Carpenter was a Robert Wood Johnson Faculty Fellow in health care finance from 1991 to 1992 at Johns Hopkins University School of Public Health and Thomas Jefferson University Hospital in Philadelphia. She previously taught at the University of Minnesota from 1982 to 1989. Her research interests include the use of cost accounting data for clinical evaluations and the determinants of hospital profitability.

Barbara Goppold, RPh, BS, was formerly regional pharmacy director for Aetna Pharmacy Management (a prescription benefits management organization within Aetna health plans) in Wayne, PA. Ms. Goppold was previously the clinical pharmacy coordinator for Chestnut Hill Hospital in Philadelphia from 1981 to 1993. She has an extensive background in JCAHO (Joint Commission on Accreditation of Healthcare Organizations) and NCQA (National Committee for Quality Assurance) accreditation processes. Her publications and lectures over the last three years have included the role of managed care pharmacies in government programs, health systems integration, and disease outcomes. Ms. Goppold has served as a preceptor for a pharmacoeconomics fellowship program and is a member of the Academy of Managed Care Pharmacy, American Society of Health System Pharmacists, and other local and state organizations.

John J. Schrogie, MD, is assistant director of health policy and clinical outcomes, director of the office of clinical trials, and executive secretary of the institutional review board at Thomas Jefferson University in Philadelphia. Dr. Schrogie was trained in internal medicine and clinical pharmacology and has held positions at the Food and Drug Administration (FDA), National Institutes of Health, Schering-Plough, and Merck Research Laboratories. He founded a contract research organization, the Philadelphia Association for Clinical Trials (PACT), and served as its president and chief executive officer. Dr. Schrogie currently serves as associate secretary-treasurer of the American Society for Clinical Pharmacology and Therapeutics.

Preface

Accountability for the outcomes of health care interventions will be the watchword for the next century. This accountability includes a recognition that resources are limited and that the allocation of resources will be a necessary future challenge. Accountability also means readiness to report on the effectiveness of a health care intervention using report cards and other tools. As the health care system evolves and integrated delivery systems become responsible for the care of a patient population, accountability will be the guiding principle. Escalating health care costs result in a heightened awareness of the need to control them. At the same time, there is a realization that cost containment efforts must be combined with measures of health outcomes. One of the admirable aims of health outcomes research is to better understand how the outcomes and costs of care change as a result of different therapeutic choices. There is a growing appreciation that these types of studies can help identify unnecessary services and provide insight into the selection of cost-effective treatment regimens.

We have tried to make this book a primer that will help health care professionals understand how outcomes are an integral part of assessing the costs and consequences of health care interventions including pharmaceutical therapy. Pharmacoeconomics research is a tool in the outcomes research toolbox that helps quantitate the economic value of pharmaceuticals in the treatment of disease. A pharmacoeconomics evaluation integrates the total cost of care with the outcomes in such a way that cost–outcome ratios can be calculated and different therapeutic regimens can be compared. This type of research helps decision makers understand how the use of pharmaceuticals may change the overall costs of health care. Many pharmaceutical manufacturers, anticipating the increased demand for outcomes and pharmacoeconomic data, are increasing their budgets for economic studies to justify new high-cost, high-profile products. Many managed care organizations are seeking evidence that the use of expensive new pharmaceutical products will result in health benefits to patients and in economic benefits to health care providers. With all the interest in conducting and analyzing economic studies for these pharmaceutical products, it is interesting that few resources are available to help decision makers learn how to incorporate this information into day-to-day health care decision making. *The Role of Pharmacoeconomics in Outcomes Management* provides practical advice on how pharmacoeconomics can be incorporated into various aspects of measuring and improving patient outcomes with pharmaceuticals.

Those wishing to find ways to integrate the principles of outcomes management and pharmacoeconomics into their own practice setting can use this book. Formulary decision makers, quality management professionals, educators, and indeed, all providers, will find the book useful as it also provides a step-wise approach to turning outcomes theory into key practical applications relevant to different practice settings. This is not a textbook on the science of pharmacoeconomic methodology, but rather a guide to how pharmacoeconomics is currently used in different settings and how its role will expand in the near term.

The first three chapters provide a solid basis for understanding the development of the outcomes management field and the role that economic analysis plays in the overall scheme. Chapters 4 through 8 pay specific attention to tools and techniques that can be used to conduct and evaluate economic and outcomes analyses. The book concludes with a look at the future of outcomes assessment and a call for standardized methodology in chapter 9. We welcome your feedback and wish you luck in your work.

Chapter One

Introduction to Outcomes Management

Nelda E. Johnson, PharmD, and David B. Nash, MD

Introduction

This chapter serves as overview of the outcomes management movement and factors that fuel its development (unexplained practice variance, escalating costs, concerns about cost versus quality, and so on). Additional topics include the following:

- Use of economic analyses to measure outcomes
- Outcomes management terminology
- Health care quality and accountability (report cards)
- Application of outcomes research to pharmaceuticals assessment

The chapter lays a broad foundation for subsequent chapters built around the following issues:

- How to measure costs and outcomes
- How to incorporate results of outcomes research into formulary management activities
- How to conduct studies in a managed care environment

Forces behind the Outcomes Movement

Several factors contribute to the increased interest in assessing outcomes of health care interventions.[1] The following three are particularly significant:

1. Unexplained variation due to insufficient information about the effectiveness of common medical treatments

2. The desire to control rising health care costs
3. Concern that cost containment activities will compromise health care quality

Unexplained Variance in Health Care Practice Patterns

Research initiated more than 20 years ago has shown significant unexplained variation in the rates of various medical and surgical procedures within small geographic areas.[2-5] Key research by Wennberg found that these variations were neither associated with differences in patients' medical conditions nor resulted in different health outcomes, but rather were attributed to individual differences in physician practice styles.[6] Wennberg's research also suggested that a significant proportion of commonly used treatments did not benefit patients and represented waste in terms of health care system resources.

This concept of unexplained variations in clinical practice raised questions as to what the "best" or most effective treatments were for many medical conditions. Additional work by Dr. David Eddy showed that unexplained variations in physician practice patterns could be traced to lack of scientific evidence about the true outcomes for many health care treatments.[7,8]

Escalation of Health Care Costs

At about the same time that widespread variation in clinical practice was being recognized, concern over rapidly increasing health care costs became a major focus in the United States. Studies conducted by researchers at the RAND Corporation showed that as much as one-third of medical care provided to patients could be considered unnecessary or of little benefit.[9] As a result several groups, including the federal government, launched ambitious efforts to measure and improve the quality and effectiveness of medical care.

In 1989 Congress supported a number of new health care research initiatives and created the Agency for Health Care Policy and Research (AHCPR) to study outcomes, effectiveness, and appropriateness of health care.[10] Under the umbrella of the Public Health Service, AHCPR has overseen millions of research dollars for the study of medical effectiveness and pharmaceutical outcomes, and has developed and disseminated many clinical practice guidelines. Hopefully this type of research will make it possible to decipher what works in health care and help define care that best reflects health care consumers' needs and wants.

The Cost–Quality Relationship

The general perception that controlling or reducing health care expenditures will inevitably result in diminished quality of health care still exists in many places. However, managing health care in a targeted fashion can lower costs by emphasizing health promotion and disease prevention.

In managing patient care, it is important to focus on the cost–benefit relationship of various health care interventions and to identify the most effective treatment regimens. These elements then can be incorporated into clinical practice guidelines with the goal of reducing unwanted variance in clinical practice. Reducing the use of ineffective or unnecessary procedures can save money by allowing health care dollars to be channeled toward obtaining the best possible health outcomes.

Rationale for Measuring Outcomes

It can be said that outcomes research arose from the desire to better understand the consequences of different treatment strategies on patient outcomes. As the costs of care begin to equalize under competition pressures, however, a health care organization's quality and outcomes are likely to become key determinants in how employee benefits managers select health plans.

Some states, Iowa and Pennsylvania for example, already produce guidebooks that allow consumers to compare charges and risk-adjusted outcomes for various acute care hospitals.[11] As consumers take a more active role in their health care decisions, it will be imperative for organizations to measure outcomes that are important from the *patient's* perspective.

Three Key Definitions

Three terms—outcomes research, outcomes management, and outcomes measurement—are important to the outcomes movement. Each term is described in the following sections.

Outcomes Research

Outcomes research refers to the scientific design, data collection, and analysis of the end results of medical care. Outcomes research differs from traditional clinical trial research because it examines issues such as cost-effectiveness and the effect of treatment on quality of life. Because outcomes research strives to measure ultimate effects from the patient's point of view (such as quality of life), it does not focus solely on intermediate clinical measurements (such as laboratory tests).

Outcomes research projects are usually independent studies undertaken to evaluate the medical effectiveness of different therapeutic interventions. This type of research includes the assessment of outcomes such as changes in mortality, improvements in functional status, and satisfaction with care.

Outcomes Management

Outcomes management is a decision tool that puts the results of outcomes research studies into action. Dr. Ellwood coined the term *outcomes management* in 1988 when he described it as a "collection of patient experiences designed to help patients, payers, and providers make rational medical care-related choices based on better insight into the effect of these choices on the patient's life."[12]

Outcomes management can be considered a systematic program designed to measure and analyze patient outcomes; it is used to evaluate and improve the effectiveness and quality of the care for a particular group of patients.[13] Outcomes management extends the scope of outcomes research by using techniques similar to those applied in quality improvement programs. In some ways, an outcomes management system is analogous to a quality improvement feedback loop in which an intervention is made, data are collected, and the results (outcomes) are analyzed. Based on the results, changes are then made to the system of care to improve the overall health status of a patient population over time.[14]

Outcomes Measurement

Outcomes measurement refers to the quantitative (measurable) results of individual patient treatment as a part of routine clinical practice to assess indicators of care (such as mortality or infection rates). If the data are collected for sufficiently large numbers of patients over a period of time, these measurements can become part of an outcomes research study. If the data are pooled and used to manage and systematically improve the health care of a group of patients, the initiative could be considered an outcomes management program.

Quality and Accountability in Health Care

Health care organization accrediting entities, including the Joint Commission on Accreditation of Healthcare Organizations (JCAHO) and the National Committee for Quality Assurance (NCQA), are keenly interested in health care outcomes. The same can be said of those who pay for medical care — such as state and federal governments, insurers, and employers.

Many organizations are implementing practice guidelines and using outcomes research results to set policy and formulate criteria for performance measurements. For instance, some organizations measure physician conformance to well-accepted published guidelines and provide incentives or rewards for providers that deliver high-quality, cost-effective care. With accreditation organizations focusing their evaluation criteria on patient outcomes, it is likely that the drive to measure, manage, and improve patient outcomes will increase.

Report Cards

Many business leaders, third-party payers, and policy makers believe that the use of practice guidelines will reduce the amount of unnecessary or inappropriate medical care. Guideline compliance may form the basis for *report cards* that summarize the results of outcomes evaluations. Health care purchasers can then use these report cards as a means to select health care plans for their members or employees.

A number of managed care organizations have already developed report cards that are available to both business and consumer groups to help them compare and select health care plans.[15] These report cards can be seen as a movement toward differentiating health care organizations on the basis of quality of care and selected patient outcomes.

Outcomes Research as Applied to Pharmaceuticals Assessment

A survey of hospital pharmacists conducted in the early 1990s revealed that 88 percent of respondents felt that there was a need for more information about how to evaluate existing outcomes research, as well as a need for more pharmaceuticals-related outcomes studies.[16]

Indeed, one could view pharmacoeconomics as a key outcomes management tool. Pharmacoeconomics goes beyond basic clinical trials of efficacy (Does the therapy work in the ideal setting of a controlled clinical trial?) to effectiveness and efficiency (Does the product work in the real world and at what total cost to a health care organization?). The tools of pharmacoeconomics enable policy makers to understand the true total costs of drug therapy and, conversely, true costs of the lack of appropriate drug therapy. In this way, those responsible for formulary budgets can broaden their analysis of pharmaceutical products and focus on the total impact of drug costs.

In addition, formulary committees are now looking at patient-focused outcomes measures (such as quality of life) before making decisions. With third-party payers assuming more authority for drug purchases, pharmaceutical companies now need proof that their drugs offer a range of benefits, including better cost-effectiveness ratios and better medium-term or long-term improvements in clinical outcomes or quality of life.[17] Outcomes research is one way in which this type of information can be made available to formulary decision makers.

Outcomes research for pharmaceutical products can be conducted as part of a prospective study or by analyzing data contained in administrative or clinical databases. One fundamental component of this type of research is the use of severity-of-illness measures to adjust for differences in patients' clinical conditions.[18] This facilitates the comparison of drugs used in clinical practice outside the framework of a random controlled clinical trial. As such, these case mix adjustment systems broaden the applicability of pharmacoeconomics.

Conclusion

As providers and payers attempt to contain health care expenditures while maintaining the desired quality of health care services, we have entered an era where analyzing the effectiveness, costs, and outcomes of medical interventions has gained importance. This chapter described the outcomes movement's evolution and demonstrated how results can be a useful tool for measuring quality and pharmaceutical outcomes. Such analyses are useful to the health care organization both internally and externally:

- *Internally* to compare and select competing therapies including pharmaceutical products and to measure and improve patient outcomes through use of guidelines and feedback measurements
- *Externally* to market services to purchasers and allow customers and regulators to evaluate the organization's level of quality

The remainder of this book provides details on how costs and outcomes can be measured and how results of pharmacoeconomic studies can be used in the formulary decision-making process.

References

1. U.S. Congress, Office of Technology Assessment. *Identifying Health Technologies That Work: Searching for Evidence.* Chapter 2: Behind the search for evidence. Publication no. OTA-H-608, Washington, DC: U.S. Government Printing Office, Sept. 1994.

2. U.S. Congress, Office of Technology Assessment.

3. Wennberg, J. E., Freeman, J. L., Shelton, R. M., and Bubolz, T. A. Hospital use and mortality among Medicare beneficiaries in Boston

and New Haven. *New England Journal of Medicine* 321:1168–73, 1989.

4. Chassin, M. R., Brook, R. H., Park, R. E., and others. Variations in the use of medical and surgical services by the Medicare population. *New England Journal of Medicine* 314(5):285–90, 1986.

5. Wennberg, J. E. The paradox of appropriate care. *Journal of the American Medical Association* 258:2568–69, 1987.

6. Wennberg, J. E. Dealing with medical practice variations: a proposal for action. *Health Affairs* 3:6–32, 1984.

7. Brook, R., Kamberg, C., Mayer-Oakes, A., and others. *Appropriateness of Acute Medical Care for the Elderly: An Analysis of the Literature.* Santa Monica, CA: RAND Corporation, 1989.

8. Ellwood, P. M. Outcomes management: a technology of patient experiences. Shattuck Lecture. *New England Journal of Medicine* 318(23):1549–56, 1988.

9. Study of Patient Outcomes Associated with Pharmaceutical Therapy. AHCPR Grant Announcement. Washington, DC: U.S. Department of Health and Human Services, Public Health Service, Mar. 1992.

10. U.S. Congress. New projects funded. Research activities, Agency for Health Care Policy and Research. U.S. Department of Health and Human Services, Public Health Service. Washington, DC: U.S. Government Printing Office, 161:6–7, 1993.

11. Kenkel, P. Hospitals. *Business and Health Magazine* 13(Suppl C):19–23, 1995.

12. Ellwood, P. M.

13. Darby, M. Speaking the same language would benefit all. *Report on medical guidelines and outcomes research* 5:8–19, Nov. 1992.

14. Conrad, D. A. Editorial. *Frontiers of Health Services Management* 8(2):1, 1991.

15. Winslow, R. Report card on quality and efficiency of HMOs may provide a model for others. *The Wall Street Journal*, Mar. 9, 1993, p. B.1.

16. Anonymous. Hospital outcomes study signals need for research. *Health Care Financing Review* 14:215, 1992.

17. Glass, H. E. Formulary listings and the quality of life. *Script Magazine* Vol. 38, 1995.

18. Markson, L., Nash, D., Louis, D., and Gonnella, J. Clinical outcomes management and disease staging. *Evaluation and the Health Professions* 14(3):201–27, 1991.

Chapter Two

Outcomes Assessment

John J. Schrogie, MD

Introduction

As the end result in the process of delivering health care products and services to patients, outcomes should be used to measure changes in health status. They can be used for several purposes, for example:

- To evaluate effectiveness of health care interventions
- To support and understand research conclusions
- To measure health care system accountability
- To provide an information basis on which improvements in health care treatments can be assessed

This chapter details various types of measurable outcomes such as clinical results of therapy, effects on patients' health status and satisfaction levels, quality of life, and costs associated with care delivery. Additional topics include the following:

- Use of outcomes data
- Outcomes assessment criteria
- How different practice settings affect outcomes measurement considerations

Types of Outcomes Measured

The types of outcomes usually measured can be grouped into three general categories:[1]

1. *System-centered clinical outcomes:* This category includes factors that reflect the clinical results and performance of therapeutic

interventions, services, and products provided by health care professionals and the process or system for delivering that care.

2. *Patient-centered outcomes:* These include factors that reflect the effect a therapeutic product or service has on how patients perceive their health status and satisfaction with care. The category includes quality of life parameters.

3. *Cost outcomes:* This category encompasses the use of resources (financial, human, materials, support) associated with application of a product or service in a health care system.

Each category, along with specific outcomes that can be measured, is explained in the following sections.

System-Centered Clinical Outcomes

Clinical outcomes, which reflect the physiologic effects a product or service has on the patient, are the outcomes best understood by most health care providers. Measures of clinical outcomes reflect the expected or intended effect of the therapeutic intervention, where actual delivery or use of the intervention is assumed. In other words, when the clinical results of a medication are measured the patient is assumed to have complied with instructions for taking the medication.

These measures generally depend on accuracy of the original methods for measuring efficacy (such as microbiologic or clinical cures for patients with pneumonia) and the performance and quality of the health care system in which care is delivered. It should be noted that many of the measures traditionally used for medications — especially those that lower cholesterol, blood glucose, or blood pressure — are deemed to be *surrogate endpoints* that simply represent the agent's immediate pharmacological effect. To accurately measure a drug's *long-term clinical outcome,* changes in rates of morbidity, mortality, or complications must be assessed.

In addition to the clinical outcomes described above, other factors may be considered as evidence of the quality and outcomes of clinical care *as well as* the effects of an organization's care processes or systems. For example:

- Unanticipated return to surgery to correct results of an unsatisfactory intervention
- Nosocomial infections due to inadequate infection control procedures
- Iatrogenic complications introduced by the provider during the course of treatment
- Adverse effects from drugs or devices

- Management of disabling clinical symptoms such as pain or psychological distress
- Rates of rehospitalization, outpatient visits, or emergency procedures subsequent to medical treatment

Assessment of clinical outcomes, then, is really a reflection of several factors:

- Performance of individual health care providers
- Process of care within the health care system
- Ability of treatments to achieve clinically desirable therapeutic ends or to avoid undesirable consequences

Patient-Centered Outcomes

Several types of outcomes measure the patient's perception of his or her functional health status, quality of life, or satisfaction with care. These measures are discussed below.

Functional Health Status

Measuring a patient's functional status assesses the effect that a therapy or service has on the patient's ability to perform usual daily activities at home or at work. Until recently, relatively little attention was paid to this area of measurement. A notable exception is rehabilitation medicine, which concentrates on measuring patients' response to therapy by applying criteria that are meaningful to patients (assessment of physical functions such as walking, eating, or dressing, for example).

A patient's functional status also may be routinely assessed following orthopedic surgery for hip procedures. In all cases, measures of functional response to therapy are best assessed directly by the patient rather than indirectly by outside experts, including health care professionals.[2-4]

Quality of Life

The World Health Organization has defined the phrase *quality of life* as "a state of complete physical, mental and social well-being, and not merely the absence of disease or infirmity."[5] Measuring quality of life involves assessing how patients perceive and react to their health status and to the *nonmedical* aspects of life (ability to earn income, for example).

In clinical situations the more specific term, *health-related quality of life*, is used, a designation that is value-laden. For example, certain aspects of life (freedom from life-style restrictions, enjoyment of environmental quality) are not directly related to an individual's health.[6,7] Health-related quality of life is detailed at length in a later section.

Satisfaction with Care

Another patient-centered outcomes measure assesses patients' satisfaction with the health care services and procedures they received. With the delivery of care being moved from single-visit provider encounters to population-based managed care methods, increased emphasis is placed on using business models (for example surveys) to evaluate customer satisfaction. Individual managed care organizations must now compete based on such satisfaction ratings of their systems' care delivery.

Thus, report cards are more commonplace as patient surveys assess their satisfaction levels. These assessments evaluate provider performance, which in turn affects decision making and provides the basis for marketing the organization's services.

Performance reports, however, provide only limited information about the quality of health care. Many managed care program administrators regularly survey their providers' performance using certain parameters:

- Waiting time to obtain a physician appointment
- The scheduler's timeliness and courtesy when addressing the appointment request
- Condition of the waiting facility
- Whether the patient was evaluated according to schedule
- Whether information was provided to improve patient's understanding of his or her condition and the treatment plan
- Whether efforts were made to enhance patient compliance with the treatment regimen

Ongoing study of these and other such performance factors as potential criteria for quality and patient satisfaction is critical.

Health-Related Quality of Life

In caring for patients, physicians usually focus on aspects of health-related quality of life (HRQoL). If a patient is severely ill, however, it is reasonable to assume that almost any aspect of his or her life can be affected by the health status.[8]

Because of the value individuals attach to various life aspects, patients may have secondary or indirect interest in the clinical outcomes measured, because these frequently are perceived to be under the physician's control. Thus, clinical parameters may not correlate proportionately with the patient's functional capacity and well-being, which have more direct interest and familiarity for patients. For example, a patient with severe chronic pulmonary disease might have satisfactory laboratory test results (a clinical measure), but the results may correlate poorly with his or her desire to carry out normal daily activities such as walking without assistance (a values-based measure).

Another reason to assess HRQoL is to measure patients' individual response to therapy. That patients with similar clinical measurements may have dramatically different responses to therapy is a common observation. For example:

- Patient X may suffer side effects from medications that dramatically reduce HRQoL, while patient Y tolerates the side effects quite well.
- Patients X and Y, both with severe pulmonary restriction, may have varying capacity to perform daily work and, consequently, different levels of emotional well-being.
- Patient X may continue working throughout major episodes of depression, while patient Y (also diagnosed with clinical depression) may leave work and suffer diminished well-being as a result of becoming less productive.
- Chronically ill patients may regard a brief stay in the hospital as little more than a modest distraction before returning to a relatively sedentary life at home due to illness.

Selection and Use of an HRQoL Questionnaire

Literally hundreds of HRQoL indexes have been developed. Selecting which HRQoL to use depends on several factors:

- Purpose of the study
- Clinical condition and treatments evaluated
- Validity and reliability of the questionnaire
- Ease of administering and scoring the questionnaire

Three questions must be answered before administering an HRQoL questionnaire.

Is a Generic or Disease-Specific Questionnaire Appropriate?

This question addresses the relative benefits between a generic questionnaire that assesses a wide range of health aspects (such as the Short Form 36, or SF-36) and one that is more specific to a particular disease (such as the Functional Living Index-Cancer, or FLIC). In some cases, both types may be useful, one to measure overall health status, the other to measure patients' perceptions of specific disease-related conditions. It may be appropriate for several questionnaires to be used together in a battery to obtain a comprehensive picture of the impact of different interventions on HRQoL.

Generic instruments frequently measure the following aspects, or domains, of health status:

- General health perception
- Physical functioning
- Mental health
- Social and role functioning

Disease-specific instruments are more sensitive to the clinical condition of interest and therefore may detect unique aspects, such as:

- Differences in treatment regimens
- Side effects of drugs

No matter which type of instrument is selected, only those questionnaires with proven reliability and validity in the patient population of interest should be considered. Developing a new questionnaire may not be advisable because it takes years and considerable expertise in the field of psychometrics to construct and test a valid and reliable instrument.

How Will the Information Be Collected?

Considerations here include the following:

- *Who will provide information?* Studies have shown that patients provide the most reliable answers, contrasted to health care providers answering the questions for the patients.
- *When will the questionnaire be administered?* Questionnaires can be administered at baseline and then at periodic intervals to assess response to treatment over time. The SF-36 is designed to be administered at least at four-week intervals.
- *How will the questionnaire be administered?* Questionnaires can be administered in the physician's office, mailed to patients, or administered over the phone.

How Will Changes Be Evaluated?

A decision must be made for how to interpret changes in patients' HRQoL once questionnaires are completed. Following are two examples of how this might be done:

- Compare changes in HRQoL for individual patients over time, and change the therapeutic regimen to optimize their HRQoL.
- Assess HRQoL for a group of patients to compare the effects of different treatment regimens.

Cost Outcomes

Cost or economic outcomes reflect those finance-related resources needed to provide health care service and products to patients. Cost outcomes have been particularly useful in evaluating the cost–benefit relationship of health care technologies, procedures, and products.

The assessment of cost outcomes in relationship to other outcomes (such as quality of life and clinical outcomes) can be made using the tools of pharmacoeconomics. By linking together the outcomes produced with the costs required to produce those outcomes, pharmacoeconomics helps define the relationship between the cost of a product or service and the consequence produced. Considerations in assessing cost outcomes include the following:

- What are the costs of an intervention across all the various components of an integrated health care system? Cost outcomes should measure the total cost of care, not just the costs for one component such as pharmaceutical costs.
- What are the unit costs, or resources, associated with producing a successful clinical or patient outcome for a service or product?
- What are the incremental or additional costs of delivering a particular product or service, compared with other products or services?

Cost outcomes can be obtained from a number of sources. Additional details on assessing costs and using pharmacoeconomic methodologies are found in chapter 4.

Uses of Outcomes Data

Outcomes measures can be used for a number of purposes, including the following:

- *New product development:* Traditionally, new product development at pharmaceutical companies has been limited to demonstrations of clinical safety and efficacy in random clinical trials. Now, new measures such as HRQoL outcomes are being extended to research that includes results of demonstrated clinical effectiveness derived from observing new products used in actual clinical practice, rather than under conditions of close protocol control.

- *Rationale for purchasing decisions:* Given the escalating concerns about medical care costs, outcomes information has been requested both by payers for the products and services and by patients who receive them to justify purchasing decisions. Assessments of value include determination of how well the product actually performed (quality), and whether the effects produced (outcomes) are useful to the patient, payer, or provider of care.[9]
- *Changes to therapeutic regimens:* Providers can establish a foundation for making changes to therapy protocols. By establishing treatment and disease prevalence trends, population demographics, or clinical or formulary guidelines, outcomes can be measured against standards, and clinical results can be managed.[10,11]

Identification of Outcomes Assessment Parameters

Outcomes information can be derived from a wide variety of sources, the selection of which depends on need for, and availability of, the data. Linkages between data sources for clinical, cost, and quality of life outcomes are not generally available and the methods to create these relationships often must be specially created. Following are seven parameters around which outcomes assessment systems can be planned:

1. *Time course of an illness:* Is the condition acute or chronic?
2. *Length of disease episode:* What is the time from onset to cure, recurrence, or temporary resolution?
3. *Perspective of the study:* To whom is the outcomes measurement important?
   - Payer—HMO, indemnity plan?
   - Provider—individual physician group, institution, pharmacist, nurse?
   - Patient—who assesses health status and manifests satisfaction levels?
4. *Methods of data collection:*
   - Retrospective chart review raises questions of completeness, accuracy, validity, and includes outpatient office records as well as inpatient charts.
   - Prospective studies must consider size, duration, calculation of statistical power, whether to add to an ongoing clinical trial, ability to conduct longitudinal research, and inclusion

of protocol-driven costs. A major benefit here is the ability to select exactly which parameters are studied.

5. *Data sources:*
   - Large databases include billing or claims sources, electronic medical record. On the other hand, they also raise questions of accuracy, validity, completeness, and whether sources are retrospective or prospective and can be conducted longitudinally. They also must distinguish between whether cost or charge information is available.
   - Interviews
     - Patient interviews can use direct questionnaires, report cards, or surveys.
     - Provider interviews can determine clinical care profiles.
6. *Data linkages:*
   - These encompass methods to identify patients through disease registries and create linkages to clinical records. For example, oncology patients can be identified through tumor registries; other clinical patients can be identified through chart review. Once patients are identified, they may be linked through their medical record number to a hospital information system for additional cost and resource utilization information.
7. *Availability of funds to support study:*
   - Generally speaking, retrospective chart review and linkage studies are the least expensive and fastest to perform. They are useful in building decision models or decision trees and provide the basis for designing prospective studies. On an intermediate level of expense and difficulty, the evaluation of large databases and patient interviews may be ranked. The most expensive and difficult studies to perform are large-scale prospective studies.

Some items in health care organizations are convenient to measure but reflect the *process* of health care and do not have a direct relationship to actual patient outcomes or quality of service. Such items — rates of immunizations and mammograms, for example — are not particularly useful. Therefore, other elements should be measured that are more directly linked to significant quality endpoints and patient outcomes (such as survival rates after a CABG procedure).

Providing timely data with minimal expense and without a burden to those responsible for conducting the analysis is difficult. Morbidity and rare but significant complications of care are hard to assess, particularly at the level of the individual physician, where small numbers hamper evaluation of many aspects of care, and variations in patient risk and disease severity may be considerable. Also, appropriate data linking the selected outcome indicators with quality of care should be developed.

As the evaluation of products and services shifts from a compartmentalized approach to cost containment to a more systemwide assessment of the economic effects on other portions of the health care delivery system (such as hospital readmissions due to treatment failures), significant opportunities exist to conduct outcomes assessment. Similarly, when considering the provision of services, outcomes evaluations may extend for the entire episode of illness beginning with an onset, perhaps at home, and include visits to a professional office, then to a hospital, and extend to a long-term care or hospice facility. Thus, course of illness is tracked to some point, either cure or resolution, as an intermediate endpoint.

The Managed Care Setting

As health care delivery is restructured, it is increasingly important that the system be managed on a business basis in order to ensure financial viability. To be able to measure outcomes, a managed care organization must have access to a database and to clinical guidelines to measure actual performance against a standard. A major goal of measuring outcomes in managed care is to identify outliers in product services or costs and thereby reduce variability. Managed care organizations must be committed to supporting the costs of data acquisition and making them available for their own management purposes.[12]

Rates of preventive services and specific procedures (for example, a mammogram, flu vaccines, cesarean sections) are receiving attention as potential indexes of quality of managed care. It should be remembered, however, that procedure rates are a measure of process rather than outcome. Nevertheless, rate data are relatively easy to collect in that much of them are available on computerized databases. Although rate studies are easier to conduct than outcome studies, they have major drawbacks:

- They measure only the process of care, which is related to its outcome only in an indirect way.
- Because they are based on cross-sectional rather than longitudinal data, they provide no insight on what happens to particular patients as a result of treatments received.
- A change in enrollment status can be a problem because without specific identifiers there is no way to determine what happens to patients who change enrollment for job-related or other reasons.

A variety of endpoints can be used effectively by managed care organizations to measure quality of performance. For example:

- Hospital readmission rates for particular diagnoses or illnesses
- Low birth weight incidence, although this has not been directly related to any quality indexes
- Services per episode for selected diagnoses; that is, the number of office visits, diagnostic procedures, or other interventions that are required or provided for particular diagnoses
- Patient satisfaction as described previously
- Number of office visits
- Hospital length of stay
- Compliance with drug therapy (numerous studies document the cost of filling prescriptions through benefits programs, but achievement of less-than-desirable effects due to failure to use the drug or comply with directions is not often reported)
- The provision of home health care as an alternative to hospitalization
- The provision of hospice care as an alternative to institutionalization
- The specialty versus primary care provider mix
- Measurements of the population's life-style in a particular organization, compared with the performance of groups in other locations
- Determination of whether a particular group is predisposed to particular diseases for genetic or environmental reasons
- Resource utilization management among the relatively few patients who represent a disproportionate expense — improvement of which is the focus of many outcomes studies

Most important, outcomes measures can identify gaps in communication with providers. These measures can also identify problems in the drug delivery system itself, which might be manifested by a non-return for a prescription refill or physician visit because the system functioned improperly. Analyses such as these enable managed care pharmacy providers to improve the quality and efficiency of pharmacy networks and throughout the drug delivery system.

Managed Care Data Sources

Different data sources will be used in different settings. In many staff model health maintenance organizations (HMOs), for example, there are no claims data. In fee-for-service settings where patients may see multiple physicians, complete data from medical charts are difficult to obtain. Even among health plans that maintain claims-based payment, there is wide variation in coding, the frequency with which records are updated, and the procedures used to assure quality.[13]

The Health Plan Employer Data and Information Set (HEDIS), developed by the National Committee for Quality Assurance (NCQA), is a prominent effort to provide performance reports for health plans. It is expected that managed care plans will incorporate performance measures into their quality improvement programs.

The current version of the NCQA report card, HEDIS 2.5, includes more than 60 performance indicators covering quality, access to and satisfaction with care, membership and use of services, finance, and management. The influence of HEDIS is reflected in the results of a recent national survey of 108 managed care plans, 80 percent of which claimed to have reviewed HEDIS as a model for quality assessment.[14]

Many health plans have begun to recruit populations with special health care needs (such as those covered by Medicare or Medicaid). Measures to assess the quality of care will need to be adapted to populations with different life-style practices or predisposition to certain illnesses. Further, many managed care plans lack experience in meeting the special needs of elderly and poor patients.

The Hospital Setting

Changes in resource utilization produced by the introduction of new products or services provide a good opportunity for measuring outcomes in the hospital setting.[15,16] These changes may lead to changes in treatment methods (decreased morbidity from use of intravenous solutions) or diagnosis (more precise and timely) that, in turn, lead to beneficial changes in the outcomes produced. Six potential resource utilization changes include the following:

1. New interventions might change the use of diagnostic procedures.
2. Performance of laboratory work might change from a centralized location to the bedside.
3. Administration of a product may switch from parenteral to oral routes.
4. Time spent in the intensive care unit versus return to the floor may change.
5. The use of support devices such as infusion pumps and ventilators may be modified.
6. Staffing requirements to perform procedures may be reassessed (from nurse assistant, nurse, physician resident, to attending physician).

In many hospitals, sophisticated tracking of resource utilization (room use, personnel utilization, pharmacy costs and charges, use of equipment, and procedure performance) has been developed for billing purposes as well as for support of financial negotiations with third-party payers. Unfortunately, results are rarely linked to clinical outcomes variables, and there is considerable variation in diagnostic procedures, severity-of-illness coding, and completeness of clinical progress notes.

Conclusion

Outcomes assessment is a crucial component health care institutions need to select goods and services for purchase and to evaluate the quality of clinical performance by staff and systems within the institution. These measures can also be used to assist in product development decisions and to establish the value of new products from the patient's, payer's, and provider's perspectives.

This chapter described types of outcomes that can be measured (system-centered clinical outcomes, patient-centered outcomes including patient satisfaction and HRQoL, and cost/economic outcomes) and discussed outcomes measurements as applied to the managed care and hospital settings.

References

1. National Quality of Care Forum. *Bridging the Gap Between Theory and Practice: Exploring Outcomes Management*. Chicago: Hospital Research and Educational Trust, 1994.

2. Guyatt, G. H., Feeney, D. H., and Patrick, D. L. Measuring health-related quality of life. *Annals of Internal Medicine* 118:622–29, 1993.

3. Guyatt, G. H., and Cook, D. J. Health status, quality of life and the individual. *JAMA* 272(8):630–31, 1994.

4. Gill, T. M., and Feinstein, A. R. A critical appraisal of the quality of quality of life measurements. *JAMA* 272(8):619–26, 1994.

5. World Health Organization. The first ten years of the World Health Organization. Geneva: WHO, 1985.

6. Guyatt, Feeney, and Patrick.

7. Guyatt and Cook.

8. Guyatt, Feeney, and Patrick.

9. Nash, D. B., and Markson, L. E. Managing outcomes: the perspectives of the players. *Frontiers of Health Service Management* 8(2): 3–52, 1991.

10. Johnson, N., and Nash, D. B. Incorporating outcomes into P&T activities. *Pharmacy & Therapeutics* 693–96, July 1993.

11. Gerbino, P. Maximizing therapeutic outcomes through cost-effective formulary decisions. *Managed Healthcare Pharmacy* 31–36, 1994.

12. Lewis, B. E. HMO outcomes research: lessons from the field. *Journal of Ambulatory Care Management* 18(1):47–55, 1995.

13. Epstein, A. Performance reports on quality—prototypes, problems and prospects. *New England Journal of Medicine* 333:57–61, 1995.

14. Gold, M., Nelson, L., Lake, T., and others. Behind the curve: a critical assessment of how little is known about arrangements between managed care plans and physicians. *Medical Care Research and Review* 52(3):307–41, Sept. 1995.

15. Johnson and Nash.

16. Gerbino.

Chapter Three

Cost Measurement

Caryl E. Carpenter, PhD, and Nelda E. Johnson, PharmD

Introduction

This chapter describes different costs that may be measured, as well as their selection and data sources (for managed care and hospital environments) in an outcomes or pharmacoeconomic assessment. Other topics include the following:

- Types of hospital reimbursement methods
- Cost terminology and its relationship to the study perspective
- Determination of hospital costs used in an analysis

The chapter closes with a case study.

Types of Costs Measured

Outcomes and pharmacoeconomic evaluations can include several types of costs including the following:[1]

- *Direct medical costs,* such as payments for hospital or other medical services
- *Direct nonmedical costs,* such as transportation to a clinic for treatment
- *Indirect costs,* such as lost earnings due to illness
- *Intangible costs,* such as emotional pain and suffering

Assessing a multitude of costs is important to understanding a new drug's cost-effectiveness potential because each cost component contributes to society's overall health care costs. The costs most commonly included in economic analyses are direct medical costs, for the following reasons:

- They are the easiest costs to measure.
- They are the costs best understood by most health care decision makers.
- They have a direct financial impact on health care organizations.

In some situations, however, indirect and intangible costs might be important to an analysis when, for example, the benefits of a therapy significantly improve a person's functional status or ability to return to work. One of the challenges in conducting cost or economic outcomes assessments is deciding which costs to include.

Selection of Cost Measures

The decision as to what costs to include in an analysis will depend primarily on the methodology used for the study and the perspective, or point of view, from which the analysis is conducted.[2] For instance, if the study takes a societal perspective, then all of the above-cited costs might be important to the analysis. Yet it may not be necessary or feasible to measure all cost types in any one pharmacoeconomic analysis. In deciding which costs to include, it may be helpful to answer the following questions:

- *What are the clinical effects of the drug?* The physiological effects and intended clinical use of a drug directly influence the costs of care. For example, if using a particular drug reduces acute exacerbations of a disease and decreases hospitalization rates, then it would be important to measure direct medical costs. However, if the drug does not directly affect the medical costs but significantly improves patients' quality of life and physical functioning, it would be important to assess indirect and intangible costs.
- *What perspective will the study adopt?* The study's point of view usually will be that of the decision maker who intends to use the study results. For example, if a drug is being considered for addition to a managed care formulary, then the perspective will be that of the managed care organization (MCO). Costs incurred by the MCO (such as the amount paid out for medical and pharmacy claims) should be included in the analysis.

  If a drug will be used in the hospital, the point of view should be that of the hospital or, more specifically, a hospital administrator. If the hospital is part of an integrated health care system, then the costs of interest will be those incurred for the entire system including hospital readmissions and outpatient costs. From an employer's or patient's point of view, it would be important to assess the effect a drug has on the patient's return to work and physical functioning. Defining the study perspective is a critical factor in selecting which costs to include in an analysis.

- *What methodology will the study apply?* Frequently, the nature of the study design will dictate which costs to include in an analysis. For example, if the study will be conducted retrospectively, only those medical costs already recorded in a database will be used. Because direct nonmedical costs (such as lost time from work) and intangible costs (such as pain and suffering) usually are not elements in a medical information system, they must be measured in a prospective study; it is not possible to go back and recreate these costs. Increasingly, pharmaceutical companies are designing prospective clinical studies to provide information on the cost consequences of new therapies.

- *Is it feasible to measure the costs?* It is not always necessary or realistic to measure all cost types. For a drug that rarely causes certain severe adverse effects, it may not be necessary to measure the cost of these events if their contribution to total costs of care for a patient population is negligible. For certain types of costs (for example, costs associated with litigation) it may be difficult or cost-prohibitive to conduct a study that would identify and measure these costs. In some cases, it may be possible to obtain the needed cost information from the literature or by conducting a survey of experts in the field, rather than measuring them directly. Any costs obtained by this method should be clearly explained in the study.

Sources of Cost Data

Once the decision is made as to which costs to include in the analysis, the next step is to identify an appropriate data source from which to obtain the costs. Identification usually will depend on several factors, including:

- *The patient population and the disease or clinical condition in which the medical treatment is used:* It is always important to consider the patient population eligible to receive the treatment and whether the treatment will be administered in the hospital or in the outpatient setting. For example, if the patient population of interest will be older than age 65, it might be important to look at data for Medicare patients or to obtain data from a managed care plan whose enrollees include an elderly population. If, however, the condition of interest occurs primarily in younger patients, a managed care plan with younger members would be appropriate.

- *The perspective for the analysis:* As discussed above, the perspective used for the study lends direction in selecting the appropriate costs and data sources for the study. For example, if a pharmaceutical product is used primarily in an acute hospital setting, a study conducted from the hospital's perspective should measure actual hospital costs using data from the internal cost accounting system. It would be misleading to use patient charge data because they do not represent actual costs incurred by the hospital. From an insurer's perspective, a claims database could be accessed to determine amounts paid out for medical and pharmaceutical claims. From an employer's perspective, conducting special studies to measure lost time from work or productivity measures would be needed.

- *Data availability and access:* In that health care organizations consider their financial data to be proprietary, it is necessary to obtain permission to access medical cost data. Some organizations are more willing than others to share their financial data for the purpose of conducting health economic studies. For patient-specific cost data such as lost time from work, it may be necessary to obtain patients' informed consent if data are being collected solely for research purposes.

- *Study resources:* Using large databases such as those available for Medicare and Medicaid patients usually requires significant time and effort. It also requires computer programming skills and statistical and data analysis resources. Because these resources require adequate funding and personnel, they are not usually used by formulary decision makers and other health care providers but by health care researchers that have received large grants. A more practical approach to obtaining medical cost data is to access the data directly from hospitals or managed care organizations. There are several advantages and disadvantages to using provider cost data.
  - *Advantages:* Patient-specific details about clinical diagnoses and treatments are usually available. Study results may be more applicable to the formulary decision maker.
  - *Disadvantages:* The sample size may be too small if data from only one health care organization are available. Costs among health care organizations may differ significantly.

Types of Managed Care Cost Data

Ideally, a pharmacoeconomics analysis would use cost data from an organization similar to the one for which the treatment decision is being made. For example, an analysis conducted to determine the total cost of treating migraine headaches with a new medication ideally should use cost data obtained from an MCO whose prescription benefits program covers that medication. However, because MCO models differ (staff-model HMOs, preferred provider organizations, and IPAs, for example), it is not always feasible to conduct a study in each type of managed care setting. A study is usually conducted in one or two managed care settings so that the data can be modeled or adapted for use in other settings.

Typically, the financial data available in managed care organizations include claims submitted by health care providers for the following services:

- Pharmaceuticals
- Hospitalizations
- Primary care physician office visits
- Physician specialist visits
- Emergency department visits
- Diagnostic and laboratory tests

Each claim lists the total amount of payment requested by the provider, the amount of co-pay for which the patient was responsible, the total amount paid to the provider, and the amount of any payment denied by the managed care plan. For providers that are paid a capitated, preset amount per member per month (PMPM) for all services provided, a claim usually will not be submitted. In addition, a managed care claims database will not contain any cost data for services not covered by the plan.

Types of Hospital Cost Data and Reimbursement

It is important to understand clearly the different types of hospital financial data in order to effectively retrieve, analyze, and use the data in a cost or outcomes analysis. The types of financial data usually available in hospitals include:

- Patient charge data
- Hospital cost data
- Reimbursement data
- Utilization data

It is also necessary to understand the four methods by which providers are paid: fee for service, fee per case, per diem, and capitated payment.

Fee for Service

Historically, hospitals and other providers were paid on a fee-for-service basis whereby payment for the service corresponded to an itemized bill of charges. Payment of full charges is rare today, especially in hospitals. However, some third-party payers do negotiate to pay a percentage of the hospitals' or physicians' charges.

Fee per Case

Some third-party payers pay on a per case basis, whereby the hospital receives a set amount for each patient admission regardless of length of stay. The most familiar per case method is the federal government's diagnosis-related group (DRG) system for Medicare patients. The amount paid per hospital admission varies with the patient's diagnosis, but the amount does not vary with the number or types of services used by the patient while hospitalized.

Typically, the patient's physician sends a separate bill for professional services provided to an inpatient. Physician fees are not included in the per case rate reimbursed by Medicare. However, some payers are now "bundling" hospital and physician services into one payment for selected procedures, such as cardiac bypass surgery.

Per Diem

Under the per diem reimbursement system, hospitals receive a predetermined amount for each day that the patient is hospitalized, regardless of specific services or products received. Usually, different daily rates apply for different types of inpatient units. For example, the daily rate for the intensive care unit tends to be higher than that allowed for a routine nursing unit. The per diem method is frequently used by managed care organizations.

Capitated Payment

A capitated payment system allows for providers to receive a fixed amount per month for each plan member, regardless of whether or how many services the member actually uses. Many MCOs pay primary care physicians on a capitated basis; very few pay hospitals a capitated rate. However, some hospitals and their medical staffs have formed physician–hospital organizations (PHOs), which contract with managed care firms. The PHOs are then paid a capitated rate to provide all health care services to the members who select the PHO. In this scenario, the PHO must decide how to allocate the capitated fee to its various provider/participants.

Cost Terminology

The words *costs, charges, prices, payments,* and *expenditures* are often used interchangeably when, in fact, their intended meanings differ significantly in the context of pharmacoeconomic assessment. These distinctions are clarified in the following subsections.

Costs versus Charges

The term *costs* represents those resources used to produce a good or service. It may *cost* a hospital $1,000 to produce one day's care in a routine medical-surgical inpatient unit, but the hospital may *charge* $1,500 for this day of care. It is well established that charges for health services do not always have a consistent relationship to costs.[3]

An economic analysis that uses hospital charge data instead of actual cost data may be inaccurate and, consequently, the results useless to hospital decision makers. In a hospital, charges may be set to cover the following components:

- Actual costs of producing health care
- Losses from third-party payers, such as Medicaid, which typically pay hospitals less than actual hospital costs
- Uncompensated or indigent care
- Losses from unprofitable services, such as emergency departments
- Adjustments to provide a profit margin

In large part, a hospital's charges will depend on its payer mix. For example, consider a hospital with an average actual cost per admission of $6,000, a goal to cover its costs plus an additional 5 percent, and a payer mix as shown in table 3-1.

To calculate how much it would have to charge — charge being the unknown variable in the equation below — to recover, on average, $6,300 (the $6,000 in costs, plus an added 5 percent margin), the hospital could apply an equation for the charge: (Medicare % × Medicare payment) + (Medicaid % × Medicaid payment) + (managed care % × managed care % of charges paid) + (self-pay % × % of charges paid) = average payment, or:

$$(0.35 \times \$5,400) + (0.15 \times \$4,500) + (0.35 \times$$
$$0.80 \ charge) + (0.10 \times charge) = \$6,300$$

where: $\$1,890 + \$675 + .28charge + .10charge = \$6,300$
$\$2,565 + .38charge = \$6,300$
$.38charge = \$3,735$
$charge = \$9,829$

In this example, the average charge would have to be $9,829 (an average markup of 64 percent over costs) to receive an average of $6,300 in revenue or payments. As seen from this example, average markup depends primarily on the hospital's payer mix. However, hospitals typically assign higher markups to ancillary services such as pharmacy, laboratory, and radiology. This means that it is inappropriate to use the overall markup rate (or average cost–charge ratios) to determine the cost of a specific hospital service.

Charge and Price

The terms *charge* and *price* are synonymous. Typically, providers use the words interchangeably, whereas retailers (such as pharmacies) use the term *price* in referring to their products and services. The main difference is that "pricing" in a retail environment is more straightforward because retail pricing is usually based on a "cost plus margin" basis. Retail establishments (again, pharmacies) have not been subjected to the complicated pattern of cross-subsidization, known as cost shifting, that influences the way hospitals set charges.

Charges versus Payments

A health care provider's charges differ from *payments* received. In fact, most third-party payers do not pay the charges that providers request. Instead, they may pay according to a negotiated fee schedule, or they may pay a percentage of charges; rarely do they pay full charges.

Table 3-1. Payer Mix versus Hypothetical Payment Rate

Payer Mix	Hypothetical Payment Rate
35% Medicare	$5,400 per case on average
15% Medicaid	$4,500 per case on average
35% Managed care	Pays 80% of charges
10% Self-pay	Pays 100% of charges
5% Bad debt	Pays nothing

Expenditures and Payments

The term *expenditures* is synonymous with payments. For example, the federal government's Medicare expenditures are the payments made to health care providers (recall that these payments do not necessarily reflect either the provider's costs or charges).

For the reasons outlined in the preceding discussions, it is inaccurate to use hospital charges for a pharmacoeconomic study conducted from the hospital's perspective. If a study were conducted from third-party payer's point of view, the appropriate economic measure to include would be the amount of the payments made to the provider. It is very helpful if pharmacoeconomic analyses contain reports of the actual number of resources such as tests or procedures used, because it avoids the problem of having to decide whether to use cost or charge data and allows other organizations to use their own economic data.

Determination of Actual Hospital Costs

All hospitals have records of their charges, payments, and the costs incurred in each department; for example, what the hospital paid for salaries and supplies in the laboratory, pharmacy, and other departments. However, most hospitals have not determined the actual cost of providing a specific service or product. Many large hospitals, particularly academic health centers, have developed sophisticated cost accounting systems that allow them to determine service-specific costs.

For example, to determine the full cost of a specific drug therapy, the cost accounting system first determines actual costs incurred in each hospital department. Costs of departments that do not provide direct patient care—for example, housekeeping or administration—can be considered overhead. These costs must be allocated to all the patient care departments, including the pharmacy. Therefore, the total cost of the pharmacy becomes its direct costs plus its fair share of overhead. Next, the total number of products or services provided by the pharmacy must be determined. Finally, the cost accounting system allocates the total cost of the pharmacy (direct and overhead) to each product.

A similar process is completed for each patient care department, so the hospital can determine the actual cost of providing each service or product in the hospital. This information can then be combined with information from the billing system and medical records to determine the actual cost of each patient treated in the hospital. This kind of cost information would be readily available in most other industries but is still rare in the hospital sector.

Actual cost data for physician practices are virtually unheard of today. Most practices, at best, have records of their charges and their payments. Many practices do not even have utilization data, that is, how many services of what types were provided to their patients. Only the largest, multispecialty practices would have any kind of cost data.

Using Hospital Cost Data: A Case Example

A pharmacoeconomic analysis is being conducted for a low molecular weight heparin (LMWH) that has been shown to decrease the need for laboratory testing. If the analysis perspective is that of the hospital, financial data from the hospital cost accounting system must be accessed. A decision must be made as to which type of financial data to include in the analysis. A choice of data is available from the finance department (see table 3-2).

If the LMWH product was used for 100 hospital admissions per year, and if each patient would have received five laboratory tests during a hospitalization without the LMWH, then the hospital could have avoided a total of 500 tests per year by using the LMWH. A pharmacoeconomic analysis that used the laboratory "charge" figure in the analysis would have arrived at a result different from the one in which the hospital's direct cost was used. Even if the overhead costs were included in the analysis, the hospital would only avoid $1,335 in actual production costs by using the LMWH. An analysis that incorrectly used the charge data would have calculated that the hospital would avoid $14,000 by using the LMWH. Obviously, this would have been an inaccurate result from using the hospital's perspective. Actual hospital costs, not the amount the hospital charged to third-party payers or patients, should be used in these analyses, because charges do not accurately reflect the resources used during a hospitalization.

Conclusion

Economic and outcomes analysis may incorporate different types of costs depending on how the study is constructed and the perspective of those who will use the study results. In addition to point of view,

Table 3-2. Financial Data Choices

Direct costs for supplies and personnel to perform the test	$2.16
Allocated overhead costs	$0.51
Total costs (direct costs plus overhead costs)	$2.67
Patient charge	$28.00

it is important to know what data sources will be used and the appropriateness of cost data for the analysis.

This chapter demonstrated how these concepts apply in the process of measuring costs. It also provided examples and insight into how both perspective and methodology can influence the types of costs used in outcomes or pharmacoeconomic assessments in managed care and hospital settings.

References

1. Drummond, M. F., Stoddart, G. L., and Torrance, G. W. *Methods for the Economic Evaluation of Health Care Programmes.* Oxford, UK: Oxford Medical Publications, 1987.

2. Davidoff, A. J., and Powe, N. R. The role of perspective in defining economic measures for the evaluation of medical technology. *International Journal of Technology Assessment in Health Care* 12(1):9–21, 1996.

3. Swartz, M., Young, D. W., and Siegrist, R. The ratio of costs to charges: how good a basis for estimating costs? *Inquiry* 32:476–81, 1995.

Chapter Four

Integration of Costs and Outcomes Measurement

Nelda E. Johnson, PharmD

Introduction

Pressured by growing concerns over quality, effectiveness, and the rising cost of health care, decision makers need a method for assessing patient outcomes in relation to health care costs. This chapter describes the following methodologies:

- Ways in which economic assessments can be used in health care decisions
- Four methods for systematically assessing costs and outcomes using the tools of pharmacoeconomics

The chapter closes with a brief discussion of basic approaches and steps for using different types of pharmacoeconomic analyses.

Informed Decision Making

Economic evaluations that compare the costs of therapy to the outcomes gained can be used by health care policy makers in a number of different situations including the following:

- Development of treatment guidelines
- Pharmaceutical pricing decisions
- Formulary management decisions

Development of Treatment Guidelines

Treatment (or clinical practice) guidelines are usually developed by medical experts at the national level and then modified and adopted by health care policy makers within a health care organization. Use of economic evaluations in the development of these guidelines can have a positive effect on the costs and outcomes that result from patient care decisions. Economic evaluations can provide an important contribution in the treatment of otitis media, pneumonia, and urinary tract infections. These are conditions where the selection of a drug can directly influence the costs and outcomes. Development of cost-effective treatment guidelines can also make a significant difference for other conditions such as hypertension, peptic ulcer disease, and depression because a large number of treatment options exist for them, each with different costs, side effects, and clinical response rates.

Pharmaceutical Pricing Decisions

Decisions on what to charge for a drug therapy (or what to pay for it) can, in some cases, be based on economic evaluations that take into consideration the total treatment costs and outcomes of a therapy. For instance, a new drug might be developed by a pharmaceutical company that would decrease the number or the duration of hospitalizations, and thereby decrease the total treatment cost. This information on total treatment cost could be used as a factor in calculating a range of prices in which the drug could be determined cost-effective when compared to other treatment options.

In a similar fashion, those responsible for purchasing pharmaceutical products could conduct their own economic evaluations to determine whether a product is cost-effective. If it is not a cost-effective product (when compared to other treatments), and if lowering its price would make it a more cost-effective choice, purchasers could use this information to negotiate a price discount with the manufacturer.

Formulary Management Decisions

Formulary management decisions can contribute to improved patient outcomes and lower health care costs if those decisions are based on sound economic and outcomes data. For instance, by including on the formulary a product shown to improve patient compliance, decision makers can help reduce overall treatment costs stemming from medical complications in noncompliant patients — even if the medication costs more than other drugs in its class. Pharmacoeconomics helps answer the question "What are the additional costs that it takes to bring about improved patient outcomes?"

Some formulary managers have indicated their willingness to pay as much as 10 percent more for a drug shown to have quality of life scores that exceeded those of competitor agents.[1] How can decision makers analyze and assess the value of products that improve outcomes such as quality of life? Pharmacoeconomic analyses can help assess whether the added costs are justified, but it is necessary first to understand the overall process for selecting and using specific health economic analyses to compare costs and outcomes of the product or service being evaluated.

A 14-Step Process for Conducting Pharmacoeconomic Assessments

Health economics methodology has been adapted for use in pharmacoeconomic studies; and although it is still evolving, if used appropriately this methodology can help decision makers determine the relative value of alternative therapies. Toward this goal, Sanchez has reported a 14-step process for conducting pharmacoeconomic evaluations in health care organizations, based on published criteria for conducting health economic evaluations.[2]

- *Step 1: Define the pharmacoeconomic problem.* A clear description of the problem under consideration will help focus the study. For instance, if the problem involves comparing similar therapies that produce essentially identical outcomes, then the study should focus solely on assessing cost to purchase and use the product.
- *Step 2: Decide which perspective will be used to evaluate costs and benefits.* As explained in chapter 3, the study's point of view will be that of the health care provider, third-party payers, patients, employers, or society. Thus, a product being considered for use primarily in an acute care setting should be conducted from the hospital's perspective; if in an outpatient setting, then from the perspective of the MCO paying for the prescription and related services.
- *Step 3: Create a cross-functional project team.* A team approach will improve the likelihood of success by providing opportunity to discuss multidisciplinary use of study results. Team members might include representatives from medicine (including those who would actually prescribe the drug), nursing, pharmacy, information systems, and administration.
- *Step 4: Identify possible treatment alternatives and outcomes.* Information on potential treatment options and their outcomes can be obtained through review of the literature and through discussions with physicians. It is important to examine usual clinical practice patterns and to assess the outcomes identified by physicians within the organization as important measures of treatment success or failure.

- *Step 5: Select the appropriate pharmacoeconomic methodology.* The choice of analytical method should be based on the problem as defined in step 1. Criteria for appropriate selection of study type (including the sample criterion in step 1) are depicted in table 4-1. (Each type of economic analysis is detailed later in this chapter.)
- *Step 6: Identify resources necessary to carry out the study.* Essential resources may include access to medical records or cost data within the organization. They may also involve staff support to review literature, enter data into a database, or conduct data analysis.
- *Step 7: Assign monetary values to the outcomes.* Look at the total costs of care including labor costs, drug administration and monitoring costs, follow-up office visits, or the cost of treatment failures.
- *Step 8: Establish the probabilities of outcomes.* Refer to the range of potential outcomes identified in step 4. Outcomes data can be obtained either from published studies or, if time permits and sufficient patient population volume justifies it, an organization can conduct a study using its own data. For pharmaceutical products, common measures include efficacy rates and incidence of adverse drug effects.
- *Step 9: Use decision analysis techniques, when appropriate.* A decision tree (described in chapter 9) can help graphically illustrate the possible treatment options, their outcomes, and the costs associated with each outcome.
- *Step 10: Conduct sensitivity, marginal, and/or incremental analyses, where appropriate.* Most analyses calculate only the average cost of treatments being compared, but it is also useful to calculate the additional (or marginal) costs required to produce

Table 4-1.   Criteria for Selecting Pharmacoeconomic Study Method

Research Question for Comparing Therapies	Appropriate Method
Similar therapies producing essentially identical outcomes	Cost minimization analysis (CMA)
Different therapies resulting in clinically different patient outcomes	Cost-effectiveness analysis (CEA)
Similar therapies affecting quality of life or patient preference for treatment	Cost utility analysis (CUA)
Comparison of different programs with different outcomes (for resource allocation decisions)	Cost–benefit analysis (CBA)

one additional unit of the outcomes measure. For example, a marginal cost difference would be the extra amount spent to save one additional life by using the therapy. (Chapter 9 describes a sensitivity analysis.)

- *Step 11: Present study results to appropriate groups and professionals.* It is appropriate to present the results of pharmacoeconomic analyses to members of pharmacy and therapeutics (P&T) committees, quality improvement committees, and other professional staff who may be interested in the results because these groups use this information in their decision-making processes. They are also responsible for disseminating such information.

- *Step 12: Develop policies or clinical interventions based on study results.* Once results have been analyzed, they should be used to develop cost-effective policies for using the products or services evaluated. For example, if results demonstrate that the administration of preoperative antibiotics within two hours of surgery decreases the cost and incidence of postsurgical wound infections, hospital policies could be developed to encourage the appropriate and timely administration of prophylactic antibiotics.

- *Step 13: Implement the policy and educate others about it.* A policy implementation plan should be developed and discussed with others in the organization who may be affected by the policy (for example, nurses responsible for administering preoperative antibiotics or clerks who must notify nurses of new physician orders).

- *Step 14: Collect follow-up documentation.* Developing a plan to collect follow-up data on what impact the change exerts on patient outcomes and organization costs can help gauge program effectiveness and identify areas for improvement.

Routine and systematic collection of outcomes and cost data, along with a process for providing feedback to targeted parties, can become a part of an ongoing program to manage and improve patient outcomes within the organization.

Four Types of Economic Analyses

Four basic approaches are used to assess the costs and outcomes of pharmaceutical products and services: cost minimization, cost-effectiveness, cost–benefit, and cost utility.[3] Any one of these methods might be used in a particular study, but in some instances one approach may be more appropriate than another. It is also important to realize that not every pharmaceutical product or treatment regimen needs a full pharmaco-economic analysis. In these days of limited resources, efforts should be devoted to evaluating products that may have higher acquisition prices yet yield better patient outcomes than other available products. Table 4-2 compares the four methods, which are described more fully in the following sections.

Cost Minimization Analysis

A cost minimization analysis (CMA) compares the costs of using products shown to have very similar or identical outcomes or effectiveness rates. A common example is an assessment of the cost difference between using a brand name pharmaceutical and its generic equivalent. Because both products have the same clinical effect, it is necessary only to compare their costs and then select the lower cost agent. Cost minimization analysis may also be applied to drugs that are not generically equivalent but are considered to be therapeutically equivalent. There is little reason to devote significant efforts to complex pharmacoeconomic analyses for such products, given that the choice can be made based on drug acquisition, administration, and monitoring costs for the therapy.

Because a key assumption in a CMA is that the drugs result in similar patient outcomes, it is inappropriate to use this technique for products having different efficacy rates, different side effect profiles, or other differences that would affect outcomes. Pharmaceutical companies are not allowed to claim that a product is "cost-effective" if CMA has been used because this technique does not evaluate the product's *relative* effectiveness or outcomes, which are assumed to be equal.

Cost-Effectiveness Analysis

If the outcomes or efficacy rates of the study drugs differ significantly, then a cost-effectiveness analysis (CEA) is appropriate. This type of pharmacoeconomic evaluation compares total costs of the therapy to clinical outcomes gained. With CEA the cost elements encompass all treatment and outcomes costs—medications, laboratory and diagnostic tests, treatment of adverse drug effects, and treatment failures (the cost of managing patients who fail to respond to treatment).

A cost-effectiveness ratio (total costs ÷ clinical outcomes) is then calculated. For example, if Drug A has a success rate (outcome) of 75 percent, with total therapy costs of $1,875 per patient, the cost-effectiveness ratio would be $2,500. If, however, Drug B has an outcome of 55 percent, with total therapy costs of $605 per patient, the cost-effectiveness ratio would be $1,100, which is more desirable. In

Table 4-2. Comparison of Pharmacoeconomic Methodologies

Method	Cost Unit	Outcomes Measure	Interpreting Study Results
CMA	Dollar	Assumed to be equal	Choose product with lowest cost
CEA	Dollar	Natural clinical units (such as blood pressure)	Lowest cost per unit of effectiveness
CUA	Dollar	QUALYs or HYEs	Cost per QUALY relative to other treatments
CBA	Dollar	Dollar	Ratios of greater than 1.0

this instance, Drug B would be selected as the preferred treatment choice if the success rate or outcome is considered to be within acceptable limits.

CEA results are usually reported as the *average cost per unit of clinical outcome*. Examples of how the results might be reported include the following:

- Cost to decrease blood pressure
- Cost to prevent an episode of nausea and vomiting
- Cost per successfully treated patient
- Cost per additional life-year gained

Cost-effectiveness analyses allow decision makers to facilitate direct comparison of drugs that are used for the same clinical condition, but have different outcomes or efficacy rates. The difficulty in using these studies arises when researchers use different clinical outcomes to calculate cost-effectiveness ratios. This happens when, for instance, one researcher reports results as cost per successfully treated patient and another reports as cost per life-year gained. In this case, the ratios cannot be directly compared but stand alone as two independent analyses.

Cost Utility Analysis

A cost utility analysis (CUA) is similar to a cost-effectiveness study in that a CUA assesses total cost of therapy relative to clinical outcomes gained, but then it adjusts the outcomes measures for differences in the quality of health gained from the treatment. A CUA uses specific techniques that take into account the desirability or preferences that individuals or societies have for a particular state of health or set of health outcomes. Two techniques commonly used to assess patient preferences (also referred to as utilities) are *standard gamble* and *time trade-off* techniques.[4] Treatment options affect patient preferences for outcomes. CUAs capture the notion that people may be willing to accept a shorter life span to avoid what they perceive to be diminished quality of health due to severe disease or adverse surgical or therapeutic effects. For example, patients diagnosed with incurable cancer may prefer to undergo chemotherapy and endure months of deleterious side effects to extend their life expectancy by months or a year. Other patients may prefer not to undergo chemotherapy to have a better quality of life during their remaining time.

CUA results are most often expressed as *cost per quality-adjusted life-year* (QUALY) gained. These analyses are most often applied to medical decision making at a national level because they take the societal perspective. Until controversy is resolved with regard to how patient preferences are determined, it is unlikely that CUAs will gain widespread acceptance among formulary decision makers.

Cost–Benefit Analysis

A cost–benefit analysis (CBA) is similar to cost-effectiveness analyses in that both evaluate total costs of therapy and outcomes. However, in a CBA, outcomes (such as life-years gained) are converted to dollar values. The results are then reported as ratios expressing the relationship between costs (in dollars) and outcomes (in dollars). The advantage CBAs offer is that they allow policy makers to compare programs that have different outcomes because the outcomes measures have been converted to dollar values – unlike the clinical outcomes reported with CEA. For instance, a policy maker could determine whether it was a better investment to allocate resources to prenatal care or to a cholesterol screening program, even though these programs result in different outcomes measures. Because there is no standardized way to assign monetary values to outcomes measurement, cost–benefit analyses are more complex to conduct and are less frequently used.

Clinical Economic Studies

Although not usually considered a formal pharmacoeconomic methodology, conducting a simple cost analysis comparing different treatment regimens provides a wealth of information to health care decision makers. These studies calculate a summary measure of the net costs (or net savings) associated with different treatment regimens, services, or pharmaceutical products. This method is often preferred over formal cost–benefit analyses because the calculations are less susceptible to manipulation.[5]

The techniques of clinical economics allow health care professionals to study how different approaches to patient care influence the resources consumed in clinical medicine.[6] Sometimes these methods are referred to as *cost-offset studies* because it is possible to calculate whether the increased cost of the treatment is offset by cost savings in other parts of the health system. For example, the total cost of resources used (including medications, physician visits, hospitalizations, and emergency room care) for patients who have migraines can be measured and then compared to the total costs of care after a new, expensive drug is added to the formulary. If the new drug decreases the number of visits to the emergency room for treatment, this cost offset can be compared to the increased cost to the pharmacy for purchase of the new drug. The cost of the drug may be offset by cost reductions in other parts of the health care system. Many formulary decision makers and third-party payers find clinical cost analyses to be particularly useful because they represent the financial impact of a therapy as it is used in clinical practice.

Conclusion

Assessments that measure the total cost of treatment *relative to* outcomes gained are best for determining the overall value of pharmaceutical products. This chapter described methods by which the costs and outcomes of pharmaceuticals can be systematically assessed with pharmacoeconomic methods. Basic approaches and concepts for using different types of analyses were outlined.

References

1. Glass, H. E. Formulary listings and the quality of life. *Script Magazine* 38:45–47, 1995.
2. Sanchez, L. A. Conducting pharmacoeconomic evaluations in a hospital setting. *Hospital Pharmacy* 30:412–28, 1995.
3. Bootman, J. L., Townsend, R. J., and McGhan, W. F. *Principles of Pharmacoeconomics.* 2nd ed. Cincinnati, OH: Harvey Whitney Books, 1996.
4. Sox, H. C., Blatt, M. A., Higgins, M. C., and Marton, K. I. *Medical Decision Making.* Stoneham, MA: Butterworth-Heinemann, 1988.
5. U.S. Congress, Office of Technology Assessment. Congress of the United States. Chapter 5: The state of cost-effectiveness analysis.

In: *Identifying Health Technologies that Work: Searching for Evidence.* Publication no. OTA-H-608, Washington, DC: U.S. Government Printing Office, September 1994.

6. Eisenberg, J. M. Clinical economics: A guide to the economic analysis of clinical practice. *Journal of the American Medical Association* 262:2879–86, 1989.

Chapter Five

Disease Management Programs

Nelda E. Johnson, PharmD, and Joseph E. Biskupiak, PhD

Introduction

Many health care organizations including managed care organizations, pharmaceutical companies, and pharmacy benefits managers are pursuing disease management strategies in attempts to improve patient care and to control costs. This chapter covers the following topics:

- Definition of disease management
- How disease management, outcomes, and pharmacoeconomics are related
- Target populations for disease management programs
- Components needed to implement disease management strategies
- Key players in disease management programs
- Challenges facing program managers

What Is Disease Management?

Disease management (DM), or disease state management, is a systematic, integrated approach to managing the care of patients who have certain diseases or clinical conditions. The goal of DM programs is to improve patient outcomes while at the same time optimizing overall use of health care resources.[1] A program outlines the entire process of care for the disease state and closely aligns health care delivery steps so that optimal outcomes are achieved and resource utilization is controlled. To achieve this, DM programs must contain several components, all designed to bring together the ingredients for an integrated system of care for particular disease conditions. These components, listed below, are detailed later in the chapter.

- Patient identification process
- Clinical practice guidelines
- Patient education and participation
- Case management and intervention protocols
- Outcomes measurement and management

How Are Disease Management, Outcomes Management, and Pharmacoeconomics Related?

The goals and techniques of disease management programs bear many similarities to those of outcomes management programs. The overall objective for disease management programs is to provide cost-effective, high-quality health care for a specific patient population.[2,3] Similarly, in an outcomes management program medical treatments are selected based on economics (costs) and outcomes research, with results of care measured in terms of patient outcomes.

A disease management program, then, might be thought of as an outcomes management technique or tool designed to coordinate care for a particular disease or clinical condition. A DM program may provide more detailed information about the specific processes of patient care than an outcomes management program. This is because it not only incorporates treatment protocols, it specifies roles and activities for all health care professionals and patients along the delivery continuum. These activities are coordinated through the DM program to provide optimal patient care. Thus, program scope usually is comprehensive in that it not only seeks improved health status among a disease- or condition-specific population, but also incorporates preventive measures to maintain the health of a population that might be at high risk for the disease.

A DM program coordinates patient care activities that are designed to maximize treatment effectiveness while minimizing economic consequences of the disease. This integrated approach facilitates evaluation of total costs of care and provides an ideal opportunity to incorporate and evaluate the cost-effectiveness of pharmaceutical therapies.

The use of pharmacoeconomics to determine cost-effectiveness of drug therapy is certainly one important aspect of a disease management program. Major program efforts, however, are usually devoted to effectively integrating all aspects of care (including acute hospital care, nursing services, and home care services), not just medications. Pharmaceutical costs are not the sole consideration in a DM program; rather, cost management techniques are designed for an entire disease state, not for individual cost components of the health care system. Figure 5-1 shows how outcomes research (including pharmacoeconomics), disease

Figure 5-1.   Integrating Disease Management and Outcomes

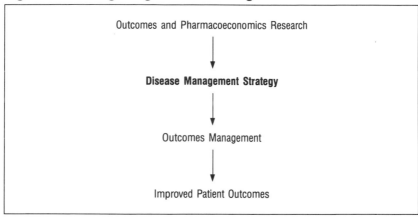

management, and outcomes management are linked to improve quality outcomes.

How Can Population Targets Be Selected for Disease Management Programs?

Although no formula serves to determine the "best" disease targets for DM programs, the most common ones are those for which it is fairly easy to measure and achieve improvements in resource utilization and clinical outcomes. Some conditions for which disease management programs have been developed are listed below:[4]

- Asthma
- Diabetes
- Heart failure
- Hypertension
- Depression
- Cancer

Most programs focus on high-cost chronic diseases such as diabetes, asthma, and heart failure, where it is expected that optimal management will result in the highest payoffs in terms of improved patient outcomes and cost control for the organization. One pilot program for patients with congestive heart failure (CHF) resulted in 60 percent fewer CHF-related hospital days, improved patient satisfaction and quality of life, and improved symptom management.[5] This pilot study had the following components:

- Early identification of clinic outpatients, before hospitalization became necessary
- Patient education materials including a video, overview booklet, and diet information sheet
- Nurse visits to patients' homes
- If necessary, provision of a scale to weigh patients
- Scheduling of regular phone appointments to monitor symptoms and answer questions

Not every disease state or clinical condition may be suitable for a disease management program. The following parameters can serve as criteria for identifying those having clinical potential for a program:[6,7]

- The disease or clinical condition is common among the health system's population.
- High-cost complications or expensive treatments are associated with the disease.
- There are unexplained variations in physicians' treatment of patients who have the condition.
- Evidence suggests that the use of clinical guidelines would improve clinical management of the disease.
- Improvements in patient compliance has been shown to be an important factor in treatment response.
- Patients with the disease can easily be identified by specific criteria.

What Are Some Components of Disease Management Programs?

Disease management programs usually encompass a number of activity components, such as those listed above. These components are further described in the following sections.

Patient Identification Process

Patient candidates for a disease management program are usually identified by virtue of their frequent hospital admissions, specialty physician visits, or emergency department visits. Using the organization's health information system is an efficient way to identify candidates, especially if the database incorporates pharmacy, medical, and laboratory data that are linked and that include diagnostic and procedure codes. They may also be identified from drug utilization reviews or through primary care physician referrals.

Clinical Practice Guidelines

A key component of DM programs is the use of clinical practice guidelines and treatment algorithms or protocols. These are used to standardize clinical management of the disease and are designed to reduce both uncertainty in medical decisions and undesirable variations in clinical practice.

Guidelines that are based on previously published, peer-reviewed documents and adapted for local use within the organization will be the most objective and effective. Published guidelines are readily available from several sources including the Agency for Health Care Policy and Research (AHCPR) and from a variety of physician specialty groups.

Patient Education and Participation

Most disease management programs include some form of patient education that stresses the importance of life-style choices, patient self-management, and medication compliance.[8] Some programs accomplish this through home health care agencies and/or visiting nurses who educate patients about their disease and how to recognize symptoms that require medical intervention.

Nurses may also provide detailed information about medication use and what effects life-style choices can have on the disease process. Patients may be given additional instructions for managing their disease and using medical equipment such as peak flow meters for asthma management or glucose monitors for diabetes management.

Case Management and Intervention Protocols

Many disease management programs use case management techniques to facilitate daily program operation. A case manager is a designated health care professional (such as a nurse manager) who coordinates patient care according to specific protocols. If symptoms indicate the need for medical assistance, the patient may be instructed first to contact a visiting nurse so that determination can be made as to what level of care is needed and where it should be delivered.

For instance, a patient with congestive heart failure may be instructed to call the case manager if there is an acute gain in weight. Based on the treatment protocol, a nurse may then administer intravenous diuretic therapy at the patient's home or in the physician's office, rather than sending the patient to the hospital. A case management approach helps manage patients more efficiently and can avoid the need for acute care hospitalizations.

Outcomes Measurement and Management

To determine the success and quality of a disease management program, patient outcomes data should be routinely measured and analyzed. Outcomes measurements may include assessments of mortality rates, hospitalization and complication rates, as well as measures of physical functioning, patient satisfaction, and health-related quality of life. In keeping with the tenets of continuous quality improvement, DM programs must be routinely evaluated and revised to update the guidelines, improve patient outcomes, and evaluate program costs.

Who Is Interested in Disease Management Programs?

The development and implementation of disease management programs may be of interest to several types of organizations:

- Health care providers
- Managed care organizations
- Large employers
- Pharmaceutical companies
- Pharmacy benefits management companies
- Disease management companies

A survey conducted by The Zitter Group (San Francisco) found that over half the MCO respondents were involved with disease management programs to some degree.[9] Recent surveys show that large employer groups are also interested in disease management programs.[10,11] As discussed next, reasons for wanting to use DM programs differ markedly among the various health care players.[12]

Health Care Providers

Providers such as large specialty clinics or physician groups may want to implement disease management programs for several reasons:

- To improve patient outcomes
- To demonstrate their capabilities in providing high-quality care in today's cost-competitive environment
- To respond to payer demands for better coordination of health care management

The latter incentive may be especially important when the provider is accountable under a capitated contractual agreement for the costs and clinical outcomes of care. Disease management programs may also be attractive to providers because, by using an efficient team-oriented approach to care, they support physicians' commitment to maintaining their patient populations' health.[13,14]

Managed Care Organizations

Disease management programs are a logical extension to MCOs as these organizations move from simply controlling resource utilization to increasing their emphasis on managing patient care, measuring outcomes, and improving the quality of health care.[15] More specifically, MCOs are developing disease management programs as an important foundation for supporting their mission of providing cost-effective health care. Many administrators are particularly attracted to the potential for cost savings and the ability to demonstrate high-quality health care. A DM program has the potential to help an organization attract new members by demonstrating a range of effective treatment options.[16]

It makes sense for MCOs to be engaged in disease management because, as the health care system matures, there is a shift away from managing individual components of health care utilization (such as pharmaceutical costs), to developing a broader perspective of what happens to patients as they move through the entire health care spectrum. However, it is important to realize that an effective DM program relies on well-integrated systems having the following features:

- Capability to identify and contact high-risk enrollees
- Ability to influence clinical treatment patterns
- Capacity to track and evaluate patient outcomes

Large Employers

Large employers who purchase health care benefits are interested in implementing DM programs primarily to improve their employees' health. A study completed in 1996 by Pinney Associates (Bethesda, Maryland) concluded that 95 percent of employers felt that their workers should be offered disease management programs.[17] In addition, a 1995 survey of employers by William M. Mercer, Inc. (Rochester, New York), found that 77 percent of respondents were likely to install an integrated DM program to help control health care costs.[18] Smoking cessation programs and other wellness programs continue to be in high demand by employers.

Pharmaceutical Companies

As pharmaceutical companies strive to demonstrate the value of their products and services to purchasers, DM programs become a viable vehicle for making their products an integral part of patient care. Many such companies are attempting to develop DM programs so as to establish partnerships with MCOs while at the same time ensuring that their products remain a part of clinical practice guidelines.

Other reasons why pharmaceutical companies want to be involved with DM programs include the following:

- To retain products on lists of reimbursed drugs
- To justify product prices
- To sell portfolios of drugs and services
- To gain competitive advantage in core businesses
- To add services and become attractive partners for customers

A pharmaceutical company with access to patient data (including prescription drug and laboratory data) is well situated to develop DM programs that can improve patient care and lower costs. However, given that most pharmaceutical companies do not have such a database, their efforts must focus on partnering with an MCO or employer.

Pharmacy Benefits Management Companies

Pharmacy benefits management companies (PBMs) are drawn to disease management programs as a means to generate additional revenue by leveraging their expertise in information systems and database development. However, without access to data such as patient medical records, a pharmacy claims database alone does not usually contain sufficient information (such as the patient's medical diagnosis) to identify patient candidates for a DM program. PBMs can certainly aid MCOs in developing and implementing disease management programs by virtue of their expertise in information systems and database development. In addition, if they have access to patient medical information, they may be successful in establishing DM programs that improve patient care through collaborative ventures.

Disease Management Companies

Some pharmaceutical companies such as Eli Lilly & Co. (Indianapolis, Indiana) and Zeneca Pharmaceuticals (Wilmington, Delaware) have established disease management units that sell fully developed programs to MCOs. Other manufacturers are developing DM protocols in collaboration with specific managed care partners.[19]

Collaborative ventures may involve pharmaceutical companies and PBMs assisting MCOs in the development of educational materials and programs for both patients and physicians. Additionally, pharmaceutical manufacturers and PBMs could assist MCOs in efforts to bolster patient compliance with medications and reinforce physician compliance with practice guidelines. Pharmaceutical companies have years of experience and knowledge about physician education and behavior modification. They can also provide MCOs with expertise acquired from years of clinical research and development and assist in designing and conducting the outcomes studies that are components of DM programs.

Challenges and Opportunities

A number of challenges and opportunities confront those who engage in activities related to disease management (pharmacy managers, formulary committee members, clinical staff, purchasers, and so on). The following list highlights only a few:

- Good outcomes research must be accessible on which to base DM program guidelines.
- Tools and data sources for measuring patient outcomes must be adequate.
- Sufficient pharmacoeconomics research must be available so that cost-effective drugs can be part of the treatment protocols.
- Data linkages must be in place to facilitate patient identification and enrollment into the program.

Conclusion

The development of disease management programs owes its popularity to the promise of improved patient outcomes at lower cost. Long-term survival as a new approach to patient care, however, will depend on ability of programs to deliver what they promise. This chapter defined disease management; described the components necessary to implement disease management strategies; and explained how disease management, outcomes, and pharmacoeconomics are related. It also cited some of the current challenges facing program planners and managers.

References

1. MacKinnon, N. J., Flagstad, M. S., Peterson, C. R., and Mesch-Beatty, K. Disease management program for asthma: baseline assessment of resource use. *American Journal of Health-System Pharmacists* 53:535–41, Mar. 1996.

2. Zitter, M. A disease-centered approach to managing pharmaceutical therapy. *Outcomes Measurement & Management* 5:1, Jan. 1994.

3. Hathaway, M. J. Managing care by managing diseases. *Managed Healthcare* S27, Oct. 1994.

4. Anonymous. New study finds DM market still immature, changing. *Disease Management News* 1(13):2-3, Apr. 1994.

5. Anonymous. HealthPartners develops clinic-based CHF program. *Disease Management News* 1(13):3, Apr. 1994.

6. Hadsalland, S. Disease management. In: S. M. Ito and S. Blackburn, editors. *A Pharmacist's Guide to Principles and Practices of Managed Care Pharmacy.* Alexandria, VA: Foundation for Managed Care Pharmacy, 1995.

7. Lumsdon, K. Disease management: The heat and headaches over retooling patient care create hard labor. *Hospitals and Health Networks* 5:34-40, Apr. 1995.

8. Ciszewski, P., editor. Demand management: a "new" strategy to solve our health care ills. *Managed Care Update* 4:6, Apr. 1995.

9. Zitter, M.

10. Anonymous. New study finds DM market still immature, changing.

11. Anonymous. Large employers look to formularies to control costs. *Managed Care Outlook* 9(8):9, Apr. 1996.

12. Short, R. Disease management: meeting the needs of different interest groups. *PharmacoEconomics & Outcomes News* 46:3-4, Jan. 1996.

13. Broshy, E., Matheson, D., and Hansen, M. Want to curb health costs? Manage the disease, not each cost component. *Medical Mark Media*, Sept. 1993, pp. 76-83.

14. Levy, R. A systems approach to cost management. *Drug Benefit Trends* 6:4-8, June 1994.

15. Special Report. Disease management: continuous health-care improvement. *Business and Health* 13:64-76, 1995.

16. Short, R.

17. Anonymous. New study finds DM market still immature, changing.

18. Anonymous. Large employers look to formularies to control costs.

19. Barnette, A. A. Strategies for the future. *Business and Health* 13(Suppl C):46, 1995.

Chapter Six

Use of Pharmacoeconomics in Formulary Decision Making

Sara J. Beis

Introduction

This chapter describes how formulary committees can use pharmacoeconomic analyses to make informed selection of cost-effective therapies. Topics include the following:

- An overview of formulary decision making
- Methods for selecting a study approach
- Ways to ensure that published data are adaptable for local use
- Guidelines for reviewing, evaluating, and validating external study results

The chapter closes with challenges and opportunities for those who are involved, or who may become involved, in the formulary decision-making process.

Overview of Formulary Decision Making

Formularies have existed in the United States since the early 1800s when they started as lists of medicinal substances for physicians to prescribe. The formulary concept became more formalized in 1959 when the American Society of Healthsystem Pharmacists (ASHP) called for new drug evaluation in the society's outline of pharmacy and therapeutics (P&T) committee activities.

Today, the formulary can be viewed as a descriptive list of pharmaceutical and biotechnology products that have been evaluated and approved by physicians, pharmacists, and other health care professionals. Products selected for inclusion are those thought to provide the highest level of efficacy and safety for an organization's patient population. Traditional formulary evaluations consisted of a thorough literature review to assess product efficacy and safety, but more recently the cost of the agent plays a bigger role in the decision-making process.

When fee for service was the primary reimbursement method for health care services, there was little incentive to control costs, especially in hospitals. But with introduction of prospective payment and hospital reimbursement at a set fee based on the patient's diagnosis — regardless of length of stay or procedures performed — hospitals initiated cost control programs. Since the mid 1980s, pharmacy departments have been viewed as cost centers, and pharmaceutical costs have become a prime target for cost containment activities.

Today, pharmacy managers are presented with a difficult budget dilemma because the cost savings achieved by reducing drug expenditures may have a direct impact not only on patient outcomes, but on medical costs in other parts of the health care system. For example, in a study published in the *New England Journal of Medicine*, investigators found that placing a cap on monthly prescription costs for New Hampshire Medicaid mental health patients reduced pharmaceutical costs but resulted in overall increases of $390,000 during the 11-month study period because visits to mental health centers and emergency departments escalated significantly.[1] It is apparent now that rational management of drug therapy costs entails ensuring an acceptable balance between assessing the safety and efficacy of pharmaceutical products while attaining economic efficiency derived from using products so that there is an *overall net benefit* to the health care system.[2]

Usefulness of Pharmacoeconomic Analyses

When pharmacy budgets are viewed as a separate, stand-alone cost item, selecting drugs that have the lowest acquisition cost may appear to be the least expensive option; however, when patient outcomes and the entire health care system are considered, products that have been shown to be cost-effective will provide the best outcomes for the system at the best cost. Thus, the evaluation of drug therapy based on the effects on overall costs and treatment outcomes has led to the development of pharmacoeconomics as a useful tool in the formulary decision-making process.

Pharmacoeconomics allows decision makers to integrate data on safety, efficacy, and overall cost of treatment to make a global assessment of the potential utility of a particular medication.[3] A pharmacoeconomic analysis assigns a value to the drug therapy, thus allowing the drug to be compared more equitably with other therapies. This does not mean, though, that pharmacoeconomic evaluations should supersede traditional evaluation of safety and efficacy data. Instead, P&T committees should use pharmacoeconomic and outcomes studies as additional tools to extend the formulary management process. Using these data helps expand that process beyond simply containing costs to optimizing drug therapy and controlling overall health care expenses.[4]

Issues to Consider before Initiating an Assessment

Before undertaking a pharmacoeconomic analysis for a formulary evaluation, several issues should be considered, as described in the following subsections, to help determine the scope and most appropriate type of economic evaluations needed.

Determine the Study Perspective

Decision makers must decide what point of view the study will take. For instance, if a product is being considered for a hospital formulary, the analysis perspective will usually be that of the hospital. If the hospital is not part of an integrated health care system, the use of outpatient cost data may not be viewed as an important component.

Conversely, for an insurance company or managed care plan that covers both inpatient and outpatient benefits, considerable value may be placed on the use of an expensive hospital drug that results in outpatient cost savings. For example, if the use of an expensive new antiplatelet agent such as abciximab (Reopro®), which is administered in the hospital during angioplasty, results in decreased hospital readmissions for repeat angioplasty and acute myocardial infarctions, this would be of particular value from the perspective of an integrated health care system.

In some cases the analysis perspective may vary within an organization, depending on the drug and who is at financial risk for the cost of care. For instance, hospitals with contractual arrangements to provide all cardiovascular services for a group of patients for a flat fee paid on a per member per month basis might take the perspective of the integrated health system or the insurance company for their pharmacoeconomic assessments.

Determine Which Pharmacoeconomic Methodology to Use

Recall from chapter 4 the four types of studies:

- *Cost minimization analyses (CMAs)*, which compare the costs of therapy for products that have the same or very similar patient outcomes
- *Cost-effectiveness analyses (CEAs)*, which assess the total cost of therapy relative to the outcomes gained, expressed as natural units (such as blood pressure)
- *Cost utility analyses (CUAs)*, which adjust the clinical outcomes for differences in the quality of health or patient preferences for health status
- *Cost–benefit analyses (CBAs)*, which convert the outcomes to dollar values so that different types of treatment programs can be compared

One example of study methodology selection is provided by the Henry Ford Health System (HFHS), an integrated system in southeastern Michigan. HFHS is a system of hospitals, physician groups, outpatient services, and a health care insurer.

The HFHS infectious diseases department discovered that certain bacteria were developing resistance to an antibiotic included on the system's formulary. As a result, department leaders requested that another antibiotic from the same class of drugs replace this agent on the list. The formulary committee selected the cost minimization method of pharmacoeconomic analysis, because the physicians considered the antibiotics in the subject drug class to be therapeutically equivalent. Had the drugs proved to result in different patient outcomes, a cost-effectiveness analysis would have been the selected method.

Review Published Studies

If a published study is available that appears to meet the committee's needs, the next step is to review the study to determine whether it is credible and whether the results are generalizable to the health care organization. If the study's cost data are inapplicable to the organization, additional data could be obtained (as explained in chapter 3). Criteria for reviewing published studies are described in the next section.

Identify Appropriate Data Sources

Data may be obtained from sources that are either external or internal to the organization. External data may be available in published literature or from product manufacturers. Medical records and cost accounting databases of the institution involved are internal data sources. In some cases a combination of data sources may be used in a cost model (see next section) to calculate the cost-effectiveness of a medication based on published outcomes or efficacy data and the organization's own cost data. The choice of data source will depend on who is conducting the study and from what perspective.

Design the Study

Once the methodology and potential data sources have been identified, the study design should be determined. Three design approaches are possible: prospective, retrospective, or modeling techniques.

Prospective Studies

The ideal scenario may be to design and conduct prospective pharmacoeconomic studies within the organization, but this requires considerable time, financial resources, and expertise. Because formulary decisions are usually made over a very short period of time (a few months), it is usually not feasible for most organizations to conduct their own prospective pharmacoeconomic studies.

Retrospective Studies

Even though retrospective studies are more easily conducted, they still take time and expertise to retrieve the data and carry out the analysis. If sufficient resources exist within the organization or through external support (such as a grant from a manufacturer or foundation), these studies can provide valuable data on costs and outcomes that accurately represent the organization's perspective and treatment patterns for the disease or clinical condition of interest.

Modeling Studies

An organization's internal financial data can be combined with clinical data from published studies to create models that show how a new drug will affect costs of care for the organization's population. For example, results from a cost model used to evaluate the pharmacoeconomic impact of therapies for prevention of deep vein thrombosis (DVT) after hip replacement surgery was recently published.[5] With this modeling technique enoxaparin, a low molecular weight heparin, was compared to the traditional, less expensive agents heparin and warfarin. Incidence data on side effects for each drug were obtained from several available literature sources; costs for the side effects were obtained from a published cost analysis; and the costs of therapy, including outpatient drug and monitoring costs, were obtained from the local health care organization that developed the model. Results of the model showed that while enoxaparin had the highest acquisition cost for the institution, it would be the most cost-effective therapy for DVT prevention among patients who underwent surgery for total hip replacement. (Creating cost models is discussed in chapter 9.) With modeling, formulary decision makers need to make sure that cost data are adaptable to their local environment.

Adapting Published Cost Data to Local Sites
Authors of the DVT economic model applied cost data from a study conducted in Canada.[6] Because authors of the Canadian study provided sufficiently detailed resource use data, the data were easily adapted for another organization's economic analysis by accessing the local facility's own cost data and making a comparative analysis. For instance, at St. John's Hospital and Medical Center (Detroit, Michigan), investigators determined the ratio of Canadian costs to local costs to be 2.6. Thus, the study's cost data were multiplied by 2.6 to give a better estimate of the local health care resource expenditures at St. John's.

Another way to adjust published cost data is by using Medicare's *resource-based relative value system* (RBRVS), developed to adjust payments for factors influencing the cost of providing medical care nationwide, including cost differences by geographic region. To adjust published cost data to local levels, determine the ratio of composite *geographic practice cost indices* (GPCI) at the study site, compared with the local GPCI value. For example, if economic data from a study conducted in Kansas City are used in Detroit, a ratio of the composite GPCI for the two cities can be compared. In Detroit the GPCI is 1.108 and in Kansas City it is 0.980. To determine the Detroit cost, the Kansas City cost must be multiplied by 1.13. Another statistic that can aid in determining differences in costs is the American Hospital Association's yearly report on the cost of beds by state and hospital size. Comparing these costs with local costs can give decision makers a general idea of cost differences between the two sites.

Guidelines for Reviewing and Evaluating Literature

Ideally, decision makers have access to sufficient numbers of published pharmacoeconomic analyses performed in environments similar to their own. Time can be well spent reviewing the literature to determine if a satisfactory study has already been conducted.

For example, when the formulary committee at the Henry Ford Health System (HFHS) evaluated varicella vaccine for inclusion on its list, they found a study on the cost-effectiveness of varicella vaccination conducted by the National Institutes of Health.[7] This study reported that the vaccination had a cost–benefit ratio of 0.9 using the *health care organization's perspective*. Because this ratio was less than 1.0, it would not be considered cost-effective from HFHS's point of view to add varicella vaccine to its formulary. However, the analysis was also conducted from the *societal perspective*, which showed significant potential benefit from using the vaccine (reductions in lost time from work). From the societal (or employer) perspective, then, the cost–benefit ratio was calculated to be 5.4, making addition of the product to HFHS's formulary a great value to its primary customers — large employers in the area.

Once a published pharmacoeconomic analysis is identified, it must be reviewed for reliability and generalizability to the organization's population. For example, if the study used clinical outcomes data obtained from randomized trials that excluded patients with comorbidities, then generalizability of the data to the population-at-large could be restricted.

Validating Published Data

Drummond and colleagues developed a comprehensive set of criteria for determining the soundness of published pharmacoeconomic studies.[8] Those criteria are summarized in the following list:

- A clearly defined research question is described.
- Analysis viewpoint or perspective is specified.
- Alternative therapy for comparison is specified.
- Evidence of the therapy's clinical effectiveness is provided.
- All relevant costs and consequences are identified.
- All costs and consequences are appropriately measured and adjusted for time.
- Additional (incremental) costs and consequences of the alternatives are provided.
- A sensitivity analysis is performed.
- Study results have been clearly interpreted.

These guidelines help sort out the *validity* of published pharmacoeconomic analyses. They are not designed, however, to assess the *usefulness* of a study for a particular health care organization.

For example, while developing an economic analysis for selective serotonin re-uptake inhibitors for treatment of depression, HFHS reviewed a published economic model for treatment of depression.[9] Although an excellent pharmacoeconomic model, the published analysis was useless to HFHS's formulary committee because instead of identifying individual drugs used in the analysis, it evaluated entire classes of drugs. Therefore, it was not specific enough to be useful in developing HFHS's pharmacoeconomic analysis.

In addition to evaluating a study's soundness, it is also important to assess other factors that help determine how applicable the study is to the decision-making organization. For example:

- *Study funding source:* Bias may be introduced if the funding source is the manufacturer of the product being studied.
- *Adaptability:* As indicated, this factor addresses whether study results are generalizable to clinical practice at the decision-making (local) organization.
- *Scope of population:* Was the study's patient population representative of patients who would receive the drug in standard local practice?
- *Comparability/control:* Was the comparator drug representative of treatment that local patients would usually receive?
- *Comparability/dosage:* Were the doses used in the study appropriate to those used in the local organization?
- *Timeliness:* Were study results available in a timely manner? If not, clinical practice standards might have changed in a way that diminishes usefulness of the study results.

Challenges and Opportunities

Those involved in formulary reviews are usually quite comfortable with assessing drug efficacy and safety data. Yet, limited familiarity with costs, patient outcome measures, and resource utilization data may inhibit their ability to assess *potential overall utility and organization-wide impact* of therapeutic agents. A few related challenges and opportunities are described below:

- Clinically trained formulary managers must become familiar with various aspects of conducting pharmacoeconomic analyses.
- Formulary reviewers must contact and network with the financial side of the organization to gain access to cost data. By approaching administrators on the common ground of ensuring cost-effective, high-quality care under new health care mandates, decision makers can be directed to key contacts in financial departments.
- Clinicians who venture into the arena of pharmacoeconomic assessment are similar to early clinical pharmacists who ventured onto the nursing units. They may be challenged by those who do not understand why clinicians are interested in financial data.

- The adventurers, who themselves may be confused by new terminology and stymied by financial methods, will be challenged to learn new ways to accomplish their tasks.
- The use of economic analyses should not stop once the formulary decision has been made. Plans for ongoing analyses should be developed to monitor and evaluate the product's true economic effect throughout the organization. Concurrent evaluations can provide further insight into the performance of a drug's use in routine clinical practice.

Conclusion

This chapter described five broad steps in the formulary decision-making process for conducting an analysis (determining the perspective, selecting the analysis method, reviewing published literature, identifying data sources, and selecting a study design). The chapter also described rationales and strategies for assessing the validity, usefulness, and adaptability of published pharmacoeconomic studies.

References

1. Soumerai, S. B., McLaughlin, T. J., Ross-Degnan, D., and others. Effects of a limit on Medicaid drug-reimbursement benefits on the use of psychotropic agents and acute mental health services by patients with schizophrenia. *New England Journal of Medicine* 331(10):650–5, Sept. 8, 1994.

2. Hatoum, H. T., and Freeman, R. A. The use of pharmacoeconomic data in formulary selection. *Topics in Hospital Pharmacy Management* 13(4):47–53, Jan. 1994.

3. Skaer, T. L. Applying pharmacoeconomic and quality-of-life measures to the formulary management process. *Hospital Formulary* 28(6):577–84, June 1993.

4. Schrogie, J. J., and Nash, D. B. Relationship between practice guidelines, formulary management, and pharmacoeconomic studies. *Topics in Hospital Pharmacy Management* 13(4):38–46, Jan. 1994.

5. Bakst, A. Pharmacoeconomics and the formulary decision-making process. *Hospital Formulary* 30(1):42–50, Jan. 1995.

6. Anderson, D. R., O'Brien, B. J., Levine, M. N., and others. Efficacy and cost of low-molecular-weight heparin compared with standard heparin for the prevention of deep vein thrombosis after total hip arthroplasty. *Annals of Internal Medicine* 119(11):1105–12, Dec. 1993.

7. Lieu, T. A., Cochi, S. L., Black, S. B., and others. Cost-effectiveness of a routine varicella vaccination program for US children. *JAMA* 271(5):375–81, Feb. 2, 1994.

8. Drummond, M. F., Stoddart, G. L., and Torrance, G. W. *Methods for the Economic Evaluation of Health Care Programmes.* Oxford, England: Oxford University Press, 1986.

9. Einarson, T. R., Arikian, S., Sweeney, S., Doyle, J. A model to evaluate the cost-effectiveness of oral therapies in the management of patients with major depressive disorders. *Clinical Therapeutics* 17(1):136–53, Jan./Feb. 1995.

Chapter Seven

Evaluation of Pharmaceutical Costs and Outcomes in Managed Care Settings

Barbara Goppold and Becky Briesacher

Introduction

In 1994 more than 50 million people in the United States were enrolled in some form of managed health care plan, representing an 11 percent increase over the previous year.[1] Results from a survey of 102 managed care organizations conducted in the early 1990s report that the primary factor ascribed to success in the managed care marketplace was "competitive pricing." Only 9 percent of respondents believed at the time that outcomes data were critical to success of the organization.

Over the next few years, as payers continue to squeeze short-term cost savings from the system (and as margins continue to decline), the priorities for health care marketplace competition are expected to change dramatically.[2] Three factors will gain in importance:

1. Measurement and use of reliable outcomes data
2. Implementation of clinical practice guidelines
3. Assessment and management of total health care costs for specific patient populations

In addition, the use of global budgets and efficiency targets will become the norm, along with incentives to provide a coordinated continuum of care as consumers and employers increasingly demand value for their health care dollars.[3]

This chapter describes how pharmaceutical benefits are managed and identifies desirable characteristics for products in a managed care formulary. It also provides a step-wise approach to assessing pharmaceutical costs and outcomes in the managed care setting. Specific topics include the following:

- Evolution of the managed care pharmacy
- Criteria for product selection
- The growing demand for outcomes studies
- The outcomes measurement process in managed care environments
- Integration of pharmacy and medical data

Evolution of Managed Care Pharmacy

Even though prescription drugs constitute only 8 to 10 percent of total health care expenditures, they offer significant potential for improved patient outcomes and cost-effectiveness. Over the past 20 years, sophisticated programs have evolved to control the cost of pharmaceutical prescriptions. Two forces driving program development are the coverage of prescription drug benefits by managed care plans, and the rapid rise in prescription drug prices.[4] Over the past four decades of managed care pharmacy evolution, prescription prices have more than doubled (see table 7-1). It is uncertain how disease management program development will affect prices by the next decade.

Many pharmacy management programs were initiated by prescription benefits management companies (PBMs) to serve as bridges for employers or MCOs offering prescription benefit plans. Although the primary function of PBMs has been to control utilization and cost of prescription drugs, this role has expanded to include the support of disease outcomes initiatives as well as research on the quality, costs, and outcomes of pharmaceutical care.[5] PBMs provide pharmacy data that vary from simplistic patient medication profiles to client–server retrieval of prescription claims. Pharmacy data have been used to develop algorithms to triage patients or determine severity of illness.

Table 7-1. Evolution of Managed Care Pharmacy

Year	Stage of Managed Care Pharmacy	Average Rx Price
1960	Prior to managed care	$3.25
1970	Prescription card programs begin	$4.00
1980	Standardized prescription claims, Mail order pharmacy, and On-line claims processing begin	$8.00
1990	Managed pharmacy programs	$25.00
2000	Disease-oriented outcomes management programs	???

Criteria for Drug Selection

Managed care providers and other large third-party payers constitute a large and growing proportion of the U.S. health care sector. They also have great potential to influence pharmaceutical prices and marketing strategies. Given the current health care environment, safety and efficacy data alone may not justify a product's appropriateness; therefore, formulary decision makers must consider a wider range of factors before accepting or rejecting a drug. As the focus shifts more toward evaluating *overall* costs and outcomes of care, managed care plans and PBMs are expected to pay for prescription drugs that meet one or more of the following criteria:

- The drug reduces the total medical costs of treating an illness.
- The product optimally improves patients' quality of life compared with other therapies.
- The product is a new therapeutic entity for the treatment of a disorder for which no other successful medication exists.
- The medication improves patient compliance, a characteristic of particular importance in conditions where missing a few doses can spell therapeutic failure.
- There is dramatic improvement in the drug's side effect profile compared with other products. Agents that reduce the need for additional medical care because of fewer clinical side effects will be advantageous.

Demand for Outcomes Studies

Many formulary committees are exploring measures such as pharmacoeconomics, improved patient outcomes, and enhanced quality of life before making decisions. Because of the increased purchasing power of PBMs and MCOs, the pharmaceuticals industry is under growing pressure to evaluate the economic consequences of their products. Although these evaluations may be initiated during the early phases of a product's clinical development, more often they are conducted after the product is already on the market. With sizable stores of computerized prescription and medical claims data on file, managed care companies and PBMs are being recognized as potentially useful sources for conducting pharmacoeconomic and drug outcomes assessment.[6,7]

A Five-Step Process for Initiating an Assessment

This section describes a sequence for assessing pharmaceutical costs and outcomes for managed care companies and PBMs. As with other evaluation initiatives, establishing a study perspective and adapting already-published data for the local environment (if necessary) are important preliminary considerations. (Review chapters 3, 4, and 5 for study point of view, methodology, and adaptability.)

Step 1: Develop a Working Hypothesis

A project hypothesis must be identified. A large managed care organization's pharmacy director who is planning an economic evaluation of nonsteroidal anti-inflammatory drugs (NSAIDs) must first develop a working hypothesis. A goal for this project might be to evaluate whether the use of a particular NSAID is associated with fewer episodes of gastrointestinal (GI) adverse effects, compared with other NSAIDs. Adverse effects to NSAIDs can result in GI ulceration and bleeding, requiring hospitalization or surgery. This side effect significantly increases health care expenditures and compromises patient outcomes. If fewer side effects were demonstrated with nabumetone, it could become the preferred NSAID, even if its acquisition price is higher. From the managed care organization's perspective, this hypothesis could be tested through a retrospective review of the medical care of members taking NSAIDs. Other elements of the study design — minimum usage of NSAIDs or exclusion of cimetidine — will determine the final analysis.

Step 2: Identify Key Costs and Outcomes

The next step is to identify what *data elements* will be used to define key costs and outcomes for the study. Data elements are components of care that make up the entire course of treatment. Continuing the example introduced in step 1, the director might define the following as important data elements:

- Number of pharmaceutical products to treat the GI side effects associated with NSAID use
- Frequency of visits to a specialist or primary care provider for GI-related complications
- Number of diagnostic tests or procedures for GI-related problems
- Number of hospitalizations or ED visits for treatment of GI complications

Step 3: Access the Study Data

Once the study has been designed, the next step is to obtain data from the organization's information system. Continuing with the example, the patient population could be identified by searching the pharmacy claims database for all patients who received NSAIDs during the time frame of interest. Obtaining pharmaceutical data for outpatient prescriptions is fairly easy because on-line claims submissions are used by most companies that provide prescription benefits. Unfortunately, pharmaceutical claims data do not usually contain clinical information, such as diagnosis or medical reason for the prescription. Consequently, it would be inappropriate to use only the prescription claims data; both the pharmacy and medical claims data must be accessed for this study.

Medical data for this patient population can be obtained by identifying all medical claims that meet the criteria specified in the study design (step 2). Specific types of medical claims can be identified by searching the database for claims with the *International Classification of Diseases* (ICD-9-CM) diagnosis codes and *Current Procedural Terminology* (CPT) codes corresponding to the outcomes of interest (both coding tools are described below). In this case, the procedures would be GI effects and GI procedures. Standardized classification systems are very useful tools for accessing diagnostic and procedural information in large databases.[8-10]

Two classification systems typically are used to identify patients with certain clinical conditions or those who received specific procedures:

- *International Classification of Diseases*, 9th revision (ICD-9-CM codes)
- *Current Procedural Terminology* (CPT codes)

Although these classification systems serve a variety of important functions, their primary use is for billing purposes. Physician offices, hospitals, insurance companies, and other health care facilities are required to provide ICD-9-CM procedure and diagnosis codes on claims submitted to Medicare. Additionally, most managed care organizations use CPT codes to track and approve payments for clinical procedures. These billing requirements have made ICD-9-CM and CPT coding a standard element in claims databases. A typical claim from a managed care database for a physician office visit might include data shown in table 7-2.

Table 7-2. Claim Form from a Sample Managed Care Database

ICD-9-CM Code	Description	CPT Code	Description	Charge	Date of Service
531.0	Gastric ulcer	432.3	Upper GI endoscopy	400.00	02May94

Step 4: Analyze the Data

Once all data have been obtained, the director must then evaluate them to determine the relationship between use of the NSAIDs and potential adverse GI effects. This means (a) looking at the time sequence of the prescription drugs relative to the medical data to determine whether the GI problems occurred after initiation of the NSAID, and (b) excluding cases where the GI disorder may have been related to another condition (such as colitis or cancer). If a relationship is found between use of the NSAIDs and GI side effects, the director may compare the total medical costs associated with these different NSAIDs.

Step 5: Interpret and Apply the Data

If costs or outcomes are better with one particular drug, it may be beneficial for the director to recommend the use of the NSAID associated with fewer adverse GI effects, even if its prescription price is higher than that of other NSAIDs. Because the goal of managing patient care is to improve patient outcomes and reduce overall costs, using a more expensive nonsteroidal product may prove beneficial in the long run.

The Outcomes Measurement Process

A guiding principle for measuring costs and outcomes in a managed care setting is to choose carefully the study components that are feasible to measure in a large population. This principle is simple to follow if the population's health status and medical care are fully documented in an integrated database. Such ideal data conditions, however, rarely exist, leaving formulary decision makers frustrated in their reliance on the limited information contained in the medical record or the information system.

The managed care organization's information system will largely determine the scope and methodology for a pharmacoeconomic study designed to assess expenditures and outcomes associated with a NSAID. In all likelihood the financial and time resources needed to conduct a large-group prospective survey of individual patients to determine their quality of life, or a manual review of patient medical charts, would be prohibitive.

For these reasons, managed care organizations often depend on automated databases rather than traditional medical chart review for defining the patterns and outcomes of pharmaceuticals use. Often these information systems have been designed to support claims processing and administrative recordkeeping functions. Although they usually contain descriptions of claims for each medical care encounter, they may not contain detailed clinical information about each member.

Integration of Pharmacy and Medical Data

In the last few years, many MCOs have begun revising their information technology capabilities with the goal of integrating all medical, laboratory, and pharmacy patient data. However, this is a labor-intensive process that requires both financial outlay and sophisticated computer programming expertise. Strengths in the following resource areas are needed to complete this goal:

- *Sophisticated in-house information technology:* Organizations need advanced computer capabilities, including relational databases and client–servers, designed to access pharmacy and medical claims data in a timely manner. (In this context, *relational databases* are those that can take the broad base of data that tracks pharmacy usage and relate it into natural groupings of information.) They may need to purchase additional software and hardware (such as a CD-ROM drive, a 2-gigabyte hard drive or larger). Client–server access via modem and appropriate support for system upkeep and service may also be required.
- *Professional expertise:* Programming professionals experienced in accessing the required data are essential. Ongoing computer software training facilitates capability to extract data from the information system using well-defined query methods developed for relational databases.
- *Estimations and acquisitions:* Although very helpful, new computerized methods of obtaining information can be expensive and time-consuming if the necessary systems have not been installed. The organization must weigh the cost of acquiring these technologies against the cost of using more traditional methods (such as chart review, which at times may have to be relied on if other systems are not yet in place). Therefore, personnel skilled in cost estimation, needs assessment, and acquisitions are crucial resources.

Challenges and Opportunities

Conducting outcomes and pharmacoeconomic evaluations challenges researchers in managed care settings to understand the limitations of their current information systems and find ways to compensate for them in the study design. Many managed care databases share several major drawbacks:[11]

- The pharmacy claims database is not routinely linked directly to the medical claims database.
- Laboratory tests results (such as cholesterol measurements) are not routinely available.
- Severity-of-illness measures are not provided as a rule.

Strategies to Ensure Study Reliability

Because the above-listed limitations are common to most managed care information systems, strategies are needed to produce valid and reliable study results. Although it will be most efficient to conduct pharmacoeconomic studies in organizations that already have an integrated pharmacy and medical database, these evaluations can still be conducted in organizations whose data are not yet integrated. Eight suggestions follow that can facilitate accurate evaluation of cost and outcomes data from managed care or PBM databases.

1. *Carefully review organizational policies.* This can ascertain whether any formulary restrictions or clinical practice guidelines might directly affect utilization of the medications under consideration. For instance, if the MCO requires prior authorization or restricts the quantity of migraine drugs dispensed per member per month, this policy could undermine a study designed to examine the economic impact of a specific drug used for migraine treatment.
2. *Review laws and regulations.* This can help identify additional restrictions and may be particularly important for external groups interested in conducting outcomes or pharmacoeconomic studies with an MCO. For example, the MCO may require measures protecting the confidentiality of certain patient populations (conditions such as AIDS or depression, for example).
3. *Fully understand the current information system that will be used to access data.* If medical and pharmacy databases are not directly linked, for example, the data must be extracted from each system and a unique member identification number, common to both systems, used to link the patient records. Typically these data are extracted and then an external data management software program (such as SAS System®, Microsoft Access® or other relational database) is used to analyze the data.

4. *Determine whether all data needed for the study are maintained on-site at the MCO or if a subcontractor manages some of the data components.* If certain programs (such as those for mental health) have been contracted out by the managed care plan (to a PBM, for example), some of these data may not be readily accessible for an outcomes analysis, in which case data extracts must be obtained from external companies. This increases the study complexity, time, and cost.

5. *Verify database accuracy before initiating data collection.* Comparing a portion of the data with a sample of medical charts can document database completeness and consistency.[12] If using claims data obtained from an external source, first verify that duplicate claims do not exist within the data extract. If they do, the data must be "cleaned" before the analysis can proceed. Someone in the organization who is familiar with the data sources can best make this assessment.

6. *Obtain a list of all data fields within the information system as soon as possible.* Samples of data elements typically found in an MCO database are shown in table 7-3. MCO or PBM personnel may have to decipher some of the data fields, especially those related to special contractual arrangements such as capitated agreements.

Table 7-3. Typical Managed Care Database Elements

Member Information	Prescription Claims	Medical Claims
Name	Drug name	Claim type
Gender	Filled date	Date of visit
Date of birth	Quantity	Diagnosis
ID number	Physician ID	Procedure
Relationship code	New/refill code	Physician ID
Dependents	Days' supply	Member status
Address	Ingredient cost	Claim amount
	Dispensing fee	Deductible
	Deductible	Co-pay
	Co-pay	Net paid out
	Net paid out	Claim number
	Pharmacy ID	
	Generic code	
	NDC code	

7. *Assess the start date of the current information system.* Doing so will help define the time frame for which data are available for analysis. For example, if the database contains claims data only for the past 18 months, a two-year study is not feasible. Although an economic assessment should identify the specific quantity of resources utilized, it is also a good idea to identify the total amount paid out for each service or claim.

8. *Create preliminary reports that contain the elements desired in a potential pharmacoeconomic study.* This is the best way to understand how data can be used and analyzed. Generally speaking, reports will include the following elements:
   - Plan type (open, closed, Medicaid, Medicare, prescription, or mental health benefits)
   - Enrollee demographics (age, gender, education, and so on)
   - Inclusive dates of enrollment for plan members
   - Disease or clinical conditions of interest (identified through ICD-9-CM codes)
   - Date of physician office visits (including primary care provider and specialist visits)
   - Date of hospitalizations and emergency room visits
   - Medical procedures (identified through CPT codes)
   - Prescription drug use (identified through national drug codes [NDCs])

Once basic data elements for the study have been selected and the preliminary reports evaluated, plans can proceed for a pharmacoeconomic or outcomes analysis in a managed care organization. Unless the MCO routinely collects information on patient satisfaction or quality of life, it will not be possible to directly analyze these types of patient outcomes without conducting a prospective survey of patients. In lieu of this, surrogate measures, or proxies (such as using laboratory values to serve as a measure for the outcomes of cholesterol-lowering medications) can be used.

Medical and pharmacy claims data from MCOs are frequently used data sources for economic outcomes analyses, especially if the study perspective is that of the third-party payer or if the drug is used primarily in the outpatient setting. Although these databases have limitations, they can serve as a rich data source for understanding the outcomes and total cost of care for different treatment regimens.

Conclusion

This chapter outlined how data from managed care companies and PBMs can be used to solve difficult decisions about balancing overall health expenditures with patient outcomes. Although a complete outcomes analysis will generally require the collection of additional information about long-term patient outcomes, a useful answer can be obtained with existing data. The preceding pages summarize guiding principles of this work and some practical considerations before initiating pharmacoeconomic projects in MCOs.

One challenge for the pharmaceuticals industry will be to provide outcomes and economic data to managed care organizations and PBMs before they make formulary decisions for their respective facilities. Provision of these data will enhance health care organizations' ability to include valuable, even if "expensive," products in their formularies.

References

1. Dimmitt, B. S. Managed care organizations. *Business and Health* 13(Suppl C):24–30, 1995.

2. Nash, D. B. Why today's health care requires integration. *Journal of Outcomes Management* 2:4–6, Fall 1995.

3. Nash.

4. Petruzzi, M. P. Evolution of managed care benefit programs. *U.S. Pharmacist* 20(7):78–86, July 1995.

5. Blissenbach, H. F. Pharmacy benefit manager: an industry in evolution. *Medical Interface* 8(10):80–88, Oct. 1995.

6. Glauber, H. S., and Brown, J. B. Use of health maintenance organization databases to study pharmacy resource usage in diabetes mellitus. *Diabetes Care* 15(7):870–76, July 1992.

7. Lohr, K. N. Use of insurance claims data in measuring quality of care. *International Journal of Technology Assessment in Health Care* 6(2):263–71, Feb. 1990.

8. Strom, B. L., Carson, J. L., Halpern, A. C., and others. Using a claims database to investigate drug-induced Stevens-Johnson syndrome. *Statistics in Medicine* 10(4):565–76, Apr. 1991.

9. U.S. Department of Health and Human Services. *International Classification of Diseases, Ninth Revision, Clinical Modification.* 4th ed. Bethesda, MD: U.S. Department of Health and Human Services, 1994.

10. American Medical Association. *Physicians' Current Procedural Terminology.* Chicago: AMA, 1994.

11. Lewis, N. H., Patwell, J. T., and Briesacher, B. A. The role of insurance claims databases in drug therapy outcomes research. *PharmacoEconomics* 4(5):323–30, May 1993.

12. Christensen, D. B., Williams, B., Goldberg, H. I., and others. Comparison of prescription and medical records in reflecting patient antihypertensive drug therapy. *Annals of Pharmacotherapy* 28(1): 99–104, Jan. 1994.

Chapter Eight

Guidelines for Conducting Pharmaceutical Outcomes Projects

Nelda E. Johnson, PharmD

Introduction

The challenge for health care workers to demonstrate that the care delivered results in better patient outcomes is of special interest for those concerned with pharmaceutical outcomes. This is because, although medications are only a small component of clinical therapy, pharmaceutical product and service choices can have direct and long-term effects on patient outcomes. This is an important fact for formulary committees to bear in mind when selecting therapies, especially given retrospective analyses suggesting that restrictive drug formularies can result in increased utilization of other health care services.[1,2]

This chapter provides practical information in the following areas:

- How and when to recognize outcomes assessment opportunities
- Ways to initiate a project
- How to organize and design a project
- How to conduct assessment initiatives
- How to report and implement results in different practice settings

Recognizing Project Opportunities

Some of the best opportunities for conducting pharmacoeconomic projects arise when changes are made in care delivery, or when new information becomes available about a drug's use. These opportunities allow providers to evaluate how changes may affect clinical and economic outcomes. Sometimes research possibilities materialize when an opportunity to improve clinical or economic outcomes is identified. Other conditions conducive to outcomes initiatives may include the following:

- New or expensive pharmaceuticals are targeted for addition to the formulary.
- Drug use evaluations identify areas for improving use of a medication.
- Published studies indicate new uses or adverse events for a medication.
- New drug use policies are implemented.
- Changes in physician prescribing patterns result from guidelines or clinical pathways.
- New pharmaceutical services are planned or implemented.

The most opportune time to conduct an analysis is when there is truly a need for the study and when it is likely that results will be put to good use. It is worthwhile to wait for and identify those opportunities, because results will be much more useful than research activities conducted simply for convenience or academic purposes.

Initiating the Project

As with many other activities, getting started can be the most difficult step of an outcomes project. Before launching an analysis, a project framework should be outlined to include a written plan that encompasses the basic elements identified by the Joint Commission on Accreditation of Healthcare Organizations (JCAHO):[3]

- Design
- Measurement
- Assessment
- Improvement

Depending on the practice setting, considerations for establishing the framework of a project might include the following:

- *Have the organization's need for, and benefits of, the project been assessed?* A study whose results primarily benefit the patient population and meet the organization's need(s) is more likely to be supported than one conducted simply because a single individual or group has a particular interest in it. For example, a project that assesses and improves pain control for cancer or surgical patients would benefit patients as well as meet the needs of a hospital that is preparing for an accreditation visit.

- *Does appropriate support exist for the project?* Securing internal support by physician groups, medical directors, or other administrators will facilitate carrying out the study and implementing changes indicated by the results. One way to engage buy-in and championship for the initiative is to present data that demonstrates that a problem or opportunity for improvement exists. If, for example, pharmacy data in a managed care plan show that members with heart failure do not receive the recommended therapy with ACE inhibitors, it would be important to discuss the data with the medical director and/or a cardiologist and ask them to champion an outcomes improvement project.

- *Are data and other resources adequate?* Data sources should be identified and evaluated for accuracy, timeliness, and appropriateness to the intent of the study. Studies requiring data extraction from multiple sources or quality of life and patient satisfaction data may require additional support (such as computer programming and data analysis skills). Availability of sufficient financial, material, and time resources also must be evaluated.

- *How will data be collected and analyzed?* Clearly outlining the study methodology not only will save time down the line, but further ensure support for the study. This is especially the case if key internal personnel have the opportunity to review and comment on the plan.

- *How will project results be communicated and implemented?* Because the results are intended to improve how the organization delivers care and services, it is important to identify ways to disseminate results internally to individuals affected by the study—reports, newsletters, or e-mail, for example. Other external ways to present results may be national conferences or publish the study in a peer review journal.

Once these and other organization-specific considerations have been settled, the work plan can be developed. A more detailed guide for implementing outcome projects is presented in the publication *A Guide to Establishing Programs for Assessing Outcomes in Clinical Settings.*[4] Although oriented toward projects conducted in hospitals, the book is general enough to be useful in other facilities as well.

Designing the Project

After selecting which condition to study, a multidisciplinary project team should be organized to design the project, set goals (including time frames for completion), and monitor progress. Initially these projects may require significant efforts devoted to obtaining buy-in of key constituents.

To facilitate successful completion, each project should be carefully designed to achieve a specific purpose within the organization. The overall purpose should be agreed upon by project team consensus, even if various components of the project may not reflect personal priority preferences of individual members. The purpose should be defined as narrowly as possible to provide a specific focus for the project, otherwise a project can become too cumbersome, and the quality of the project may suffer. A project's purpose may be as simple as evaluating the effectiveness of one treatment program compared to another for a specific medical condition.

Project design should also include appropriate protocols, data collection tools, and data analysis methods. Generally, the scope of the project defines the extent of the data collection process, the patient inclusion criteria, and the total number of patients that will be evaluated. In some cases, data collection methods may be adapted or developed from previously conducted drug use evaluations or quality improvement projects. The particular timing of the outcomes measurements and logistics for who will collect the data must be incorporated into the project's design as well.

Selection of Outcomes Measures

It is imperative to have a clear idea of the specific outcomes to be measured in the project. *Patient outcomes* can be thought of as the end result of what happens to a patient following an interaction with the health care system. As such, *outcomes measures* should reflect those patient-oriented physical and mental changes experienced by patients. In some cases outcomes may be best measured by assessing patients' physiologic response to treatment, while in other cases any changes in overall well-being or satisfaction with care should be measured.

Some processes of measuring and managing data include the following:

- *Data collection:* Complete and accurate data must be obtained— usually from patients during an encounter with the health care provider or through the mail if a follow-up survey is used. For retrospective analyses, data may be obtained from patients' medical charts or from a database. Because outcomes assessments require repeated measures over time, a system such as a special sticker on the patient's chart may be used as a reminder system.

- *Data entry:* Patient questionnaires may be bar-coded and read with an optical scanner to save data entry time. However, because this system can be an expensive investment, it is better to use a manual data entry system that can be incorporated into a clerical function. If patient-specific results are needed in a timely fashion, the data will have to be entered in real-time fashion, rather than batched for data entry at the end of the study.
- *Database management and quality control:* Data must be checked for quality control, and a back-up system must be developed to prevent loss of data due to an inadvertent error or computer malfunction. The database should be designed to check for duplicate entries and for values outside the normal or expected limits. A system for correcting any errors must also be developed and maintained throughout the study period.

The selection of specific outcomes measures most likely will depend on the clinical condition being studied and the setting in which care is provided. For example, acute care conditions may involve measuring short-term outcomes such as resolution of an acute condition, length of hospital stay, or use of health care resources during the episode. In contrast, some chronic conditions may need to be assessed by measuring patients' ability to perform activities of daily living (ADL) or by changes in their quality of life. Each outcomes measure should help assess whether the desired goal of the health care plan was achieved.

Assessing the Data

Data analysis should always be performed on a copy of the data, with the original data stored safely away. Analyses may be performed either on an individual patient basis to determine response to treatment or on an aggregate basis for the entire study population. For outcomes projects, the data analyst should be familiar with this type of data and be knowledgeable of statistical methods such as the use of multivariate analysis techniques. Interpreting data requires clinical knowledge of the variables and outcomes that have been measured. Data should be presented to personnel in a format that is readily understood; graphical representations such as bar graphs and correlation graphs are particularly helpful. Finally, discussing the results with health care providers is an essential part of developing a full understanding of how outcomes measures are linked to clinical processes such as patient treatment regimens.

Improving the Process

A plan should be developed to improve the clinical care processes using the results of the study. For instance, if one treatment regimen is clearly better than another, treatment guidelines can be developed that recommend use of the optimal treatment regimen.

Conducting the Project

Davies and colleagues described several steps for assessing outcomes in clinical settings:[5]

- Make a commitment to begin the project.
- Select a condition and organize a team for the project.
- Design the project—its purpose, scope, and data collection methods.
- Manage the data—collect, enter, and store them.
- Use the data—analyze and interpret them.

Once a commitment is made to begin measuring outcomes and a framework is in place to conduct the work, the next step is to select a specific clinical condition or procedure to evaluate. Conducting an outcomes measurement study differs from conducting traditional quality assurance activities or drug use assessments in that it evaluates all patients having a particular condition—not just those who received a specific drug or a subgroup treated by certain physicians. For example, a project designed to evaluate the outcomes of a pain management service would evaluate all eligible pain management patients, not just those who received certain medications. The advantage of the whole-population approach is that it offers opportunity to evaluate conditions and patients in which suboptimal use of medications occurs, thus identifying areas where drug therapy improvements potentially could improve outcomes.

In the early stages of conducting outcomes projects, it is best to select a condition that is relatively easy to study. The degree of difficulty in outcomes studies has been described as a function of several factors:[6]

- Potential for controversy surrounding the topic
- Type of objectives to be achieved
- Number and types of patients to be studied
- Availability of measurement tools
- Logistical and organizational complexity of the study

One way to simplify initial projects is to focus on a single diagnosis or procedure that involves only one clinical department. Later on, once expertise and support for the project have been gained, the study can be extended to include other clinical areas.

Reporting and Implementing Results

Results of an outcomes project should be presented in ways that help potential audiences clearly understand the results and then put them to good use. For *P&T committees*, this may mean using appropriate statistical tests and summarizing the data in formats similar to those used in the professional literature. For *quality improvement groups*, specific action and monitoring plans may be helpful. Any data limitations should be clearly addressed and preliminary results reviewed by clinicians before finalizing a report. Once an outcomes project is completed, results data should be combined with other activities, such as giving feedback to clinicians or installing interventions designed to improve the outcomes associated with pharmaceutical products.

Conclusion

Conducting outcomes projects for pharmaceuticals yields quantitative data on patient and economic outcomes. This information can be used to design long-term improvements in care and to assess and evaluate the effectiveness of care. Many opportunities exist for identifying and measuring patient outcomes in health care organizations. It is expected that more providers will play key roles in these projects, using the information to improve medication decisions in their respective organizations.

References

1. Sloan, F. A., Gordon, G. S., and Cocks, D. L. Hospital drug formularies and use of hospital services. *Medical Care* 31(10):851–67, Oct. 1993.

2. Horn, S., Sharkey, P., Tracey, A., Horn, C., James, L., and Goodwin, C. Intended and unintended consequences of HMO cost containment strategies: results from the managed care outcomes project. *American Journal of Managed Care* 2(3):253–64, Mar. 1996.

3. Doherty, E. C. The JCAHO agenda for change: what changes in pharmacy and in P&T activities do you need to prepare for in 1994? *Hospital Formulary* 29(1):54–68, Jan. 1994.

4. Joint Commission on Accreditation of Healthcare Organizations. *A Guide to Establishing Programs for Assessing Outcomes in Clinical Settings.* Oakbrook Terrace, IL: JCAHO, 1994.

5. Davies, A. R., Doyle, M. A., Lansky, D., and others. Outcomes assessment in clinical settings: a consensus statement on principles and best practices in project management. *Joint Commission Journal on Quality Improvement* 20(1):6–16, Jan. 1994.

6. Davies, Doyle, Lansky, and others.

Chapter Nine

Trends in Pharmacoeconomic and Outcomes Analyses

Nelda E. Johnson, PharmD

Introduction

Health care organizations are beginning to take a great interest in economic and outcomes studies. Part of organizational readiness is understanding trends and developments in pharmacoeconomic and outcomes analyses.

This chapter addresses such trends, particularly the move toward standardizing guidelines, outcomes methodology, clinical trials, and other outcomes assessment approaches. Topics include the following:

- Recognizing needs and priorities for analyses
- Standardizing pharmacoeconomic study practices
- Creating and using cost models (decision tools)
- Conducting economic analyses concurrently with clinical trials

Identifying Needs, Educating Constituents, and Prioritizing Studies

The ideal organizational setting for using pharmacoeconomics is one that is culturally and operationally attuned to the importance of cost-effective products and services. In some cases, educational programs may be required to communicate that need by clarifying what outcomes studies mean and how results can be interpreted and applied. For example, as already shown, a treatment proved to be cost-effective does not always mean that its acquisition price is lower than that of the comparator therapy.

Priorities for conducting pharmacoeconomic outcomes assessments are likely to vary depending on the organization's sophistication and what health care products or services it provides. In formulary decision making, prioritization for conducting pharmacoeconomic studies for specific medications may be ranked as either high, intermediate, or low. These categories, described in the following subsections, are illustrated in the cost–benefit decision matrix shown in figure 9-1.

High Priority

Products that cost significantly more than comparator agents but provide additional or better outcomes over less expensive products fall into the high-priority category (group II). For these drugs, economic analyses can help decision makers understand the relative value of the more expensive product and in turn help them decide whether the higher cost is worth the additional benefits gained.

Intermediate Priority

Products that are less effective and less costly than the comparator agents (group III) may also be good candidates for economic analysis, especially if their efficacy rates are within clinically acceptable limits to formulary decision makers. In some cases, these products, considered to be of intermediate assessment priority, may prove to be cost-effective in specific clinical conditions—such as in patients who need only moderate to low reductions in their cholesterol levels. Some drugs reduce cholesterol levels to a lower degree than other drugs, yet they cost less. A cost-effectiveness analysis may show these products to be cost-effective for these patients.

Low Priority

Low-priority drugs for pharmacoeconomic outcomes analysis can be split into three subcategories:

- Products that result in similar patient outcomes or have efficacy rates that are therapeutically equivalent usually do not require extensive economic analysis beyond, perhaps, cost minimization analysis. This is because purchasing decisions generally can be made based on how competitively priced the products are.
- Drugs that cost less, yet have better outcomes than comparator agents (group I on the matrix), do not require sophisticated economic analyses. They will likely be added to the formulary as a matter of course.
- Drugs that perform worse than comparator agents, yet are priced higher (group IV), will not benefit from economic analyses.

Figure 9-1. Sample Cost–Benefit Decision Matrix

	Lower Costs	Higher Costs
Higher Benefit (Increased Outcomes)	Group I. Lower cost Better effectiveness	Group II. Higher Cost Better effectiveness
Lower Benefit (Decreased Outcomes)	Group III. Lower cost Lower effectiveness	Group IV. Higher cost Lower effectiveness

Source: Johnson, N. E. A primer on pharmacoeconomics. *Journal of Outcomes Management* 2(suppl 1):8–10, 1995.

Generally speaking, these agents will not be added to the formulary even if a pharmacoeconomic analysis was conducted.

Special Needs and Priorities of Pharmaceutical Companies

Pharmaceutical companies tend to have unique needs and priorities for conducting pharmacoeconomic analyses, aside from the need to support formulary decisions. For example, they may need to determine a range of prices over which a new drug will be cost-effective as compared with alternative treatments. These companies also may have a high priority for conducting economic analyses in order to justify the pricing of their products already on the market.

Because manufacturer claims of cost-effectiveness must be supported by adequately controlled trials, it is increasingly a high priority for pharmaceutical companies to conduct economic analyses concurrently with clinical trials that will be submitted for Food and Drug Administration (FDA) approval. They also conduct economic analyses throughout the drug development process to assist with strategic research and business decisions. For example, a manufacturer may decide to discontinue development of a new product in cases where economic analyses indicate that the product will not be cost-competitive with drugs already on the market.

Developing Standardized Guidelines and Methodologies

As interest in pharmacoeconomic studies increases, so have discussions surrounding standardization of guidelines and study methodologies.

Countries that have already developed guidelines for pharmacoeconomic studies include Australia, Canada, Spain, Italy, England and Wales, and Germany. Several U.S. organizations, including the FDA and PhRMA (Pharmaceutical Research Manufacturers of America), have developed *draft guidelines*.

Obstacles to Standardization

Guidelines, including those developed in the U.S., may vary in content for several reasons:

- They may have been developed for different purposes.
- Local societal values may differ, resulting in use of varied study perspectives.
- Preferences may differ for collecting cost and outcomes data (for example, data collected in clinical trial settings versus data based on observation and meta-analyses).[1]

In Australia, where data must be submitted to the national government before a drug is covered under the national health plan, guidelines specify the use of specific cost data, types of economic data needed, and how the analysis should be carried out.

Creating and Using Cost Models

The use of cost models is becoming more frequent as researchers and pharmaceutical companies strive to provide economic evaluations to multiple audiences including different types of managed care organizations. Health care decision makers are also using cost models when published economic analyses are not available. When this is the case, it is helpful to create cost models using decision analysis techniques, such as decision trees, that facilitate structured decision making under uncertain circumstances.[2]

Decision Trees

The decision tree graphically depicts different treatment alternatives, their outcomes, and the probabilities of achieving those outcomes. Applied to pharmacoeconomics, it is a way of exploring all factors bearing on a decision in a structured fashion to determine which treatment alternative results in the best use of resources. A decision tree is shown in figure 9-2.

Figure 9-2. Sample Decision Tree

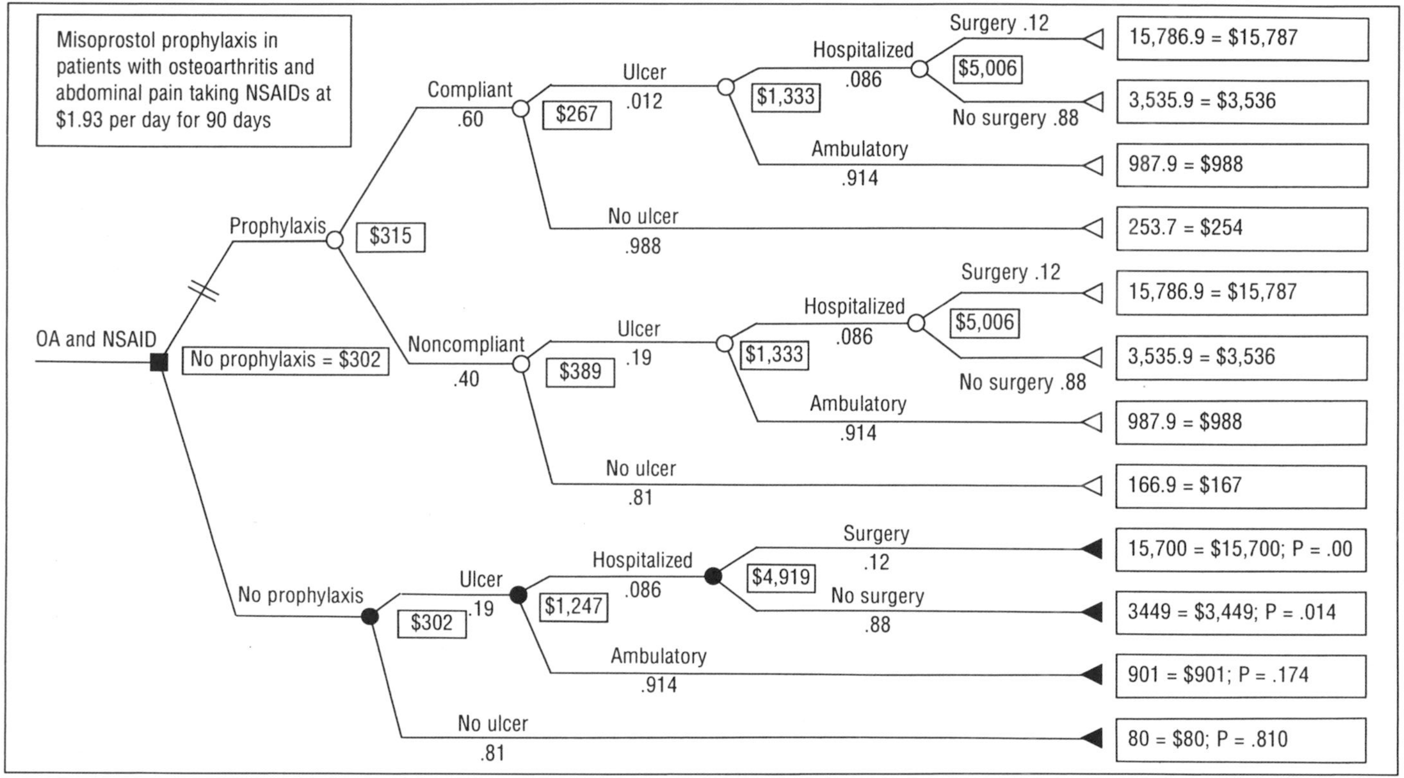

Source: Adapted from Hillman, A., and Bloom, B. Economic effects of prophylactic use of Misoprostol. *Archives of Internal Medicine*, Vol. 149, Sept. 1989.

A decision tree can help organize costs, consequences, and probabilities of each path and the possible treatment outcomes. One advantage of creating these models is that they allow decision makers to
combine their own organization's cost data with outcomes or efficacy
data from the published literature (keeping in mind the cautions regard-
ing adaptability as discussed in chapter 6). This saves time by not having to measure the outcomes. It also makes the results more applicable
to the organization. A simplified process for creating cost models using
a decision tree is outlined below. For further information, readers are
referred to additional sources.[3,4]

- *Step 1:* Visualize the possible decision choices and their outcomes. Draw the tree with each branch representing the possible outcomes attributable to each choice.
- *Step 2:* Assign the probabilities of each outcome to branches of
  the tree. Probabilities may be obtained from published clinical
  trials or outcomes studies.
- *Step 3:* Measure the costs associated with each possible outcome.
- *Step 4:* Calculate results of the model, starting at the end of the
  branches and working backward. Multiply the cost of each outcome by the probability of achieving that outcome to arrive at
  a weighted average for each branch of the tree. Continue down
  each branch of the tree, until the decision in question has been
  reached.
- *Step 5:* Interpret analysis results. The branch that results in the
  lowest weighted average cost represents the most cost-effective
  treatment choice.
- *Step 6:* Conduct a *sensitivity analysis* by varying cost data and
  efficacy data over an acceptable range of values. If the decision
  analysis results change, the model is said to be sensitive to that
  variable. For instance, if a lower price of a drug were used and
  analysis results changed, the model would be sensitive to the
  drug's price.

Several software packages are available that facilitate drawing decision trees, calculating results, and conducting sensitivity analyses. Conducting a sensitivity analysis is especially helpful with these software
packages because multiple variables can be changed and the model
recalculated to assess the robustness of the model. Software packages
useful for these purposes include the following:

- DATA: Decision Analysis by TreeAge® (TreeAge; Boston, Massa-
  chusetts)
- D-Maker (Digital Medicine; Hanover, New Hampshire)
- SMLTREE (Jim Hollenberg; New York, NY)

Using these programs can facilitate construction of a solid basis for comparing the costs and outcomes of different therapies even before a full prospective economic analysis is undertaken.

Conducting Concurrent Economic Analyses and Clinical Trials

With increased emphasis on the need to evaluate the economics of pharmaceutical therapy, pharmaceutical companies are designing and conducting economic studies alongside clinical trials. Randomized clinical trials (RCTs) are well-controlled studies designed to measure the safety and efficacy of pharmaceutical products, usually for purposes of submitting data to the FDA for product approval. As the demand for economic information has increased, economic measures of quality of life are also being incorporated into clinical trials more frequently. Certain design aspects of clinical trials, such as randomization, make them useful for comparing outcomes such as quality of life and patient satisfaction.[5]

However, because RCTs use very stringent patient enrollment criteria (patients with comorbid conditions may be excluded from a study), they may show a benefit not reproducible in the general patient population. Other problems related to conducting economic analyses as part of clinical trials include the following:[6]

- Additional protocol-driven costs (such as laboratory tests required by the study) may be introduced that would not be present in usual clinical practice.
- They may include the wrong comparators or include the use of placebo treatment which does not represent clinical practice.
- They may not include meaningful clinical endpoints useful for formulary decisions.

In contrast, economic studies attempt to measure the economic consequences of alternative treatment regimens as they are used in the "real world," such as in hospitals or managed care organizations. When economic studies are conducted as part of an RCT, they are subject to the constraints listed above. Results of these studies may not be generalizable to everyday practice. For economic analyses that are conducted during clinical trials, it is particularly important to assess several factors:

- Is the study's patient population representative of those who would receive the drug in standard clinical practice?
- Was the comparator drug representative of treatment that patients would usually receive?

- Were the study doses used appropriate to those prescribed in local clinical practice?
- How were the cost data obtained? Were standardized or estimated costs used, or were actual patient costs measured?
- Were protocol-driven costs excluded from the analysis? If patients were hospitalized just for the purpose of receiving the study drug, were these costs excluded? Were costs for any additional tests or procedures required by the protocol excluded?
- Were the study results available in a timely manner? If not, changes in clinical practice standards may diminish usefulness of the results (such as conditions formerly managed in inpatient settings now treated in outpatient settings).

To be useful, then, results from economic studies conducted as part of RCTs should meet these criteria:

- *Generalizability:* They should be consistent with usual clinical practice.
- *Timeliness:* They should be reported as quickly as feasible.
- *Site-specificity:* They should incorporate research designs that factor in the decision maker's practice setting where the drugs will be used.

Conclusion

This chapter described ways to recognize the need for, and establish priorities for, conducting pharmacoeconomic studies to support formulary decisions and validate the pharmaceuticals product development process. The trend toward standardizing guidelines and methods for economic outcomes assessments was outlined. Benefits and methods for creating cost models using decision analytic techniques were illustrated as well as the usefulness of conducting and using economic analyses concurrently with randomized clinical trials.

References

1. Jacobs, P., Bachynsky, J., and Baladi, J. A comparative review of pharmacoeconomic guidelines. *PharmacoEconomics* 8(3):182–89, Sept. 1995.

2. Barr, J. T., and Schumacher, G. E. Applying decision analysis to pharmacy management and practice decisions. *Topics in Hospital Pharmacy Management* 13(4):60–71, Jan. 1994.

3. Sox, H. C., Blatt, M. A., Higgins, M. C., and Marton, K. I. *Medical Decision Making.* Stoneham, MA: Butterworth—Heinemann, 1988.

4. Bootman, J. L., Townsend, R. J., and McGhan, W. F. *Principles of Pharmacoeconomics.* 2nd ed. Cincinnati, OH: Harvey Whitney Books Co., 1996.

5. Tsai, W., and Johnson, N. Pharmacoeconomic outcomes studies vs. randomized clinical trials. *Pharmacy & Therapeutics* 19(1):84–89, Jan. 1994.

6. Hays, R. D., Sherbourne, C. D., and Bozzette, S. A. Pharmacoeconomics and quality of life research beyond the randomized clinical trial. In: B. Spilker, editor. *Quality of Life and Pharmacoeconomics in Clinical Trials.* Philadelphia: Lippincott-Raven Publishers, 1996.

Index